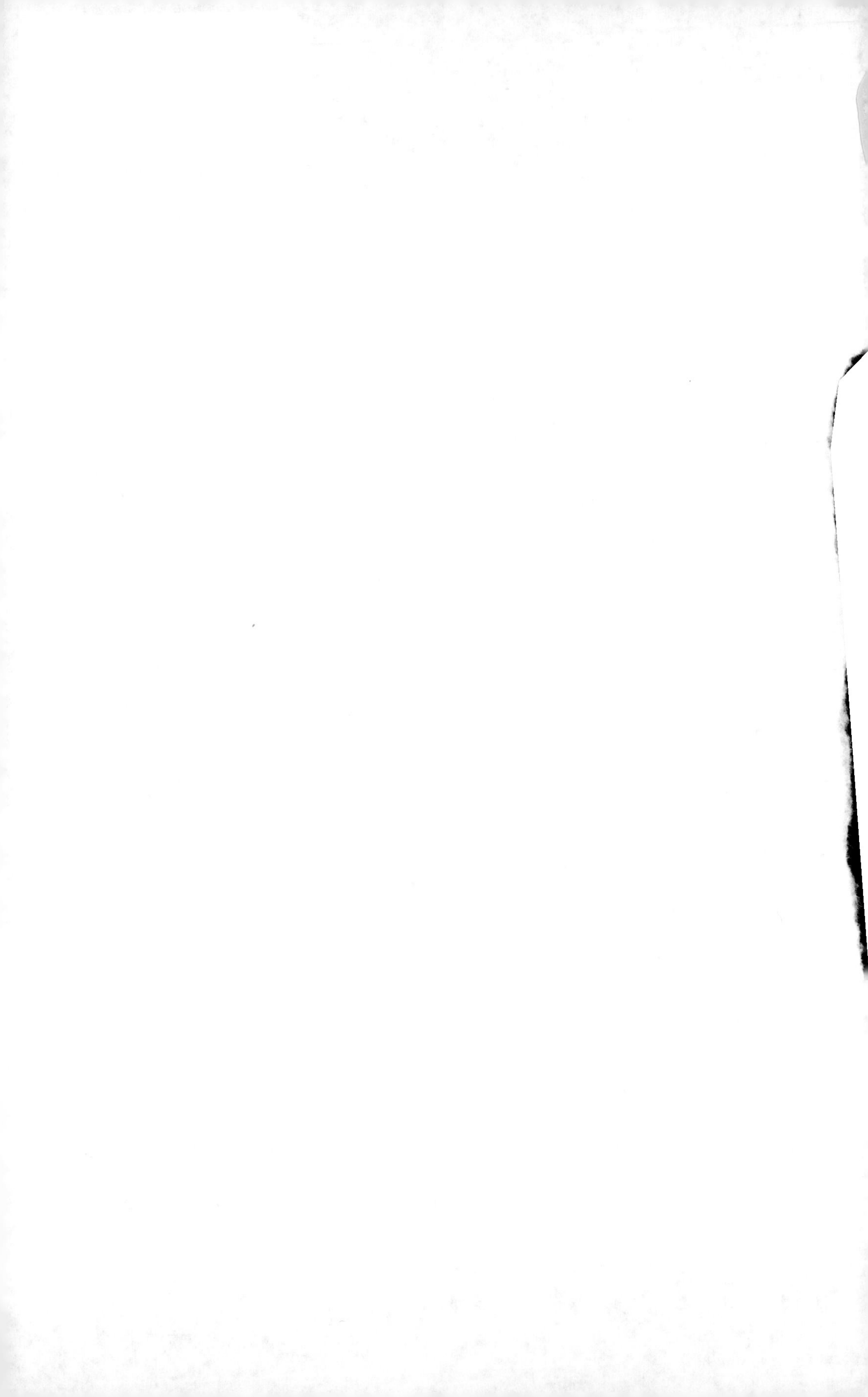

SEXUALITY AND PRISON

Emotional Despair and Constrained Desires

Arnaud Gaillard

SEXUALITY AND PRISON

Emotional Despair and Constrained Desires

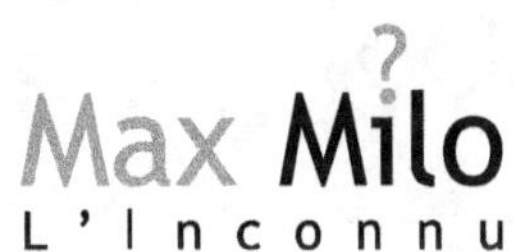

Max Milo Éditions, Paris, 2023
www.maxmilo.com
ISBN : 978-2-31501-153-7

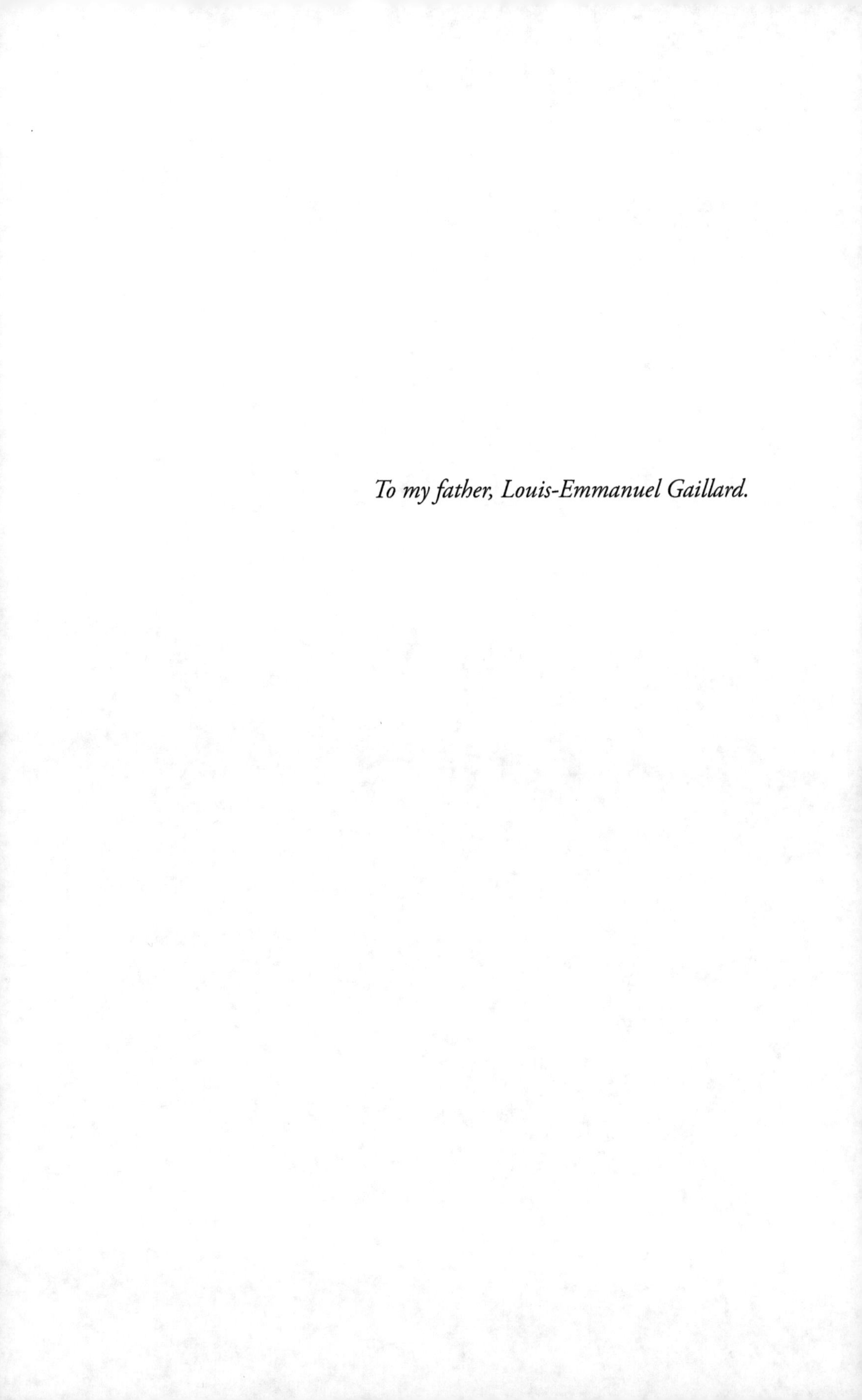

To my father, Louis-Emmanuel Gaillard.

Acknowledgements

It would be presumptuous not to include in this work those who, from near and far, have made it possible for these lines to be presented before your eyes. There is a collective element in all our reflections and challenges. For their critical eye, their encouragement, their spirit and their presence, I would particularly like to thank Danaé Bilder, Philippe Combessie, Samantha Enderlin, Eugène Enriquez, Fabrice Ferrier, Vincent de Gaulejac, Claudine Haroche, Tit-Hou Larrieu, Jacques Lesage de La Haye, Edwige Rude-Antoine, Jan Spurk and the members of RAIDH.

I'd also like to pay tribute to all those anonymous people whose confidently revealed discourse laid the foundations for an unprecedented sociological analysis.

Finally, thanks to my father, who passed on to me the pleasure of writing.

Foreword
Outside, inside

"To give a human being only what he needs is to consider him a beast.[1] According to Lear, it is precisely the satisfaction of a certain number of desires that confers the human dimension and distinguishes man from the animal species. This is also the question raised by the condition of a detained population, weaned on seduction, tenderness, chosen sexuality and shared pleasure. My major ambition was to lift the veil on the hidden intimacy of these individuals, forgotten in the shadow of impermeable walls to which protective virtues are attributed. A curiosity we'd all be wrong to accuse ourselves of.

Although prison sociology has long been considered the poor relation of contemporary research, this quest for meaning through the world-views of the inmate population informs us, through sexual issues, about the place of otherness in the construction of individuals within the social space. Symptomatically, the mechanisms of listening and trusting to *speak* in order to be *heard* represent, for these forgotten captives, a reconstitution of this missing otherness, as much on a sexual level as on a relational and social one.

---

1. SHAKESPEARE (William), *Le Roi Lear*, Paris, Flammarion, 1995.

Prison is understood here as a social universe that is both specific and, in some respects, similar to the society it represents. The individuals held there belong to the *outside world* before being confined to the *inside*. They are, or claim to be, subjects of society and actors in their own lives, in the same way as their peers at liberty. However, contingent specificities allow us to differentiate their experiences, based on the identification of a spatial rupture between outside and inside, and a temporal rupture between *before* and *after* incarceration. The monosexual universe, the punishment concealed under the constraint of bodies, the continuous surveillance, the reduced space signifying confinement, the numerous deprivations beyond even the right to come and go, the modifications to the economies of material and existential survival, the duration undergone, are all parameters that give this research a particular tone.

The process of gaining access to land cannot contradict the authority of an administration to ensure that the walls it is responsible for are watertight. The official procedure for obtaining permission to enter a French prison requires patience and obstinacy. The prison world is guarded like a seraglio. Even if the inmates know how to say, with a touch of humor: "It's harder to get out than it is to get in", the unofficial rather than the official procedure is more like an elaborate rhetoric designed to discourage curiosity. No one wanted to take on the responsibility of promoting the visibility of sexuality in detention. Prisons are meant to be closed, and the management of individuals locked up under duress must satisfy a precarious equilibrium despite the rigidity of a meticulous discipline collectively governing individual daily lives. There are exceptions to this observation, and these are the very ones that provided the gaps through which this study was nonetheless possible. The wardens who responded to our questions were also weary of the current paradox surrounding the management of sexual behavior in prisons. Between a ban on relations, based on the argument of modesty, and the provision of condoms or even Viagra, the authority of the local prison administration, the one that presides over the management of each establishment, the one that is in direct contact with the inmates, finds itself at the helm of a rudderless ship that is tending to lose all credibility. Some spoke of a legislative vagueness that is increasingly untenable in the face of inmates accustomed to the strict observance of their prerogatives, in the light of legal provisions whose ambiguities are a source of conflict and revolt. Other managers expressed an ideological as much as a pragmatic desire to promote the evolution of the experience of sexuality in terms of respect for the humanity of each individual on the one hand, and rehabilitation objectives on the other. In the end, this study was unprecedented in that it was the first sociological study of sexuality in prison to be initiated from the outside, based on empirical work carried out *in situ*.

****

Between each episode of visibility, the prison returns to the anonymity that voluntarily adorns its existence, increasingly relegated to the outskirts of cities or remote provinces whose names escape the majority of people. These are what Philippe Combessie calls "the strategies implemented to reduce the social visibility of the prison".[2] Prison exists, as a forgotten necessity in the rhythm of everyday life. Disregarding alternative sentences, it is presented as the punitive solution to which the courts give priority. Its purpose has not been freed from the ambitious theories whose limitations its analysts have been constantly accusing since its inception. And yet, prisons are a special sociological object insofar as they represent, in the secrecy of their operations, a social tool at the service of a society's overall organization. This is why a nation's

---

2. COMBESSIE (Philippe), *Prisons des villes et des campagnes*, Paris, L'Atelier, coll. "Champs pénitentiaires", 1996, p. 24.

reflection on the inescapable subject of punishment and the discharge of its debt to society undeniably leads to questions about the use and objectives of deprivation of liberty in a democratic system.

Although often defined as an irreplaceable institution, prison inspires a literature that is far from consensual. Among those who focus their analysis on this sentencing mechanism, there is a not inconsiderable proportion of inmates dealing with issues based on personal experience. Moreover, outside observers often express harsh criticism of an institution that upsets, disturbs and struggles to meet its stated objectives. In short, there is a divide, resulting from more or less radical criticism of an institution that some aspire to reform, while others condemn outright.

Before being a social tool, prison is a political tool. It represents the power of the law, the legislator and the authority of judges. It responds to imperatives of order, rights and obligations, and is part of an institutional mechanism whose fundamental questioning is beyond the scope of this study. Built on the principle of deprivation of freedom through the confinement of individuals in a monosexual universe, prisons contradict certain basic needs of the individuals in their care. Deprivation of the freedom to come and go, monosexual confinement, the difficulty of conjugal encounters, daily submission to authoritarian discipline - these are all parameters inherent to prison, which upset the ontological functioning of individuals, viewed here as socialized animals[3]. Adaptation mechanisms develop, enabling survival in this temporary universe, the outcome of which is inevitably the prospect of a new immersion in the heart of a free outside world.

---

3. On the distinction between natural desires common to men and animals, and rational desires, see THOMAS AQUINAS (Saint), *Summa Theologica*, Paris, Desclée et Cie, 1949, pp. 160-177.

Yesterday's taboos on sexuality are gradually being lifted. Whether through a psychological, sociological, physiological or even medical approach, the public debate on sexuality in prisons today requires us to reflect on this inherent aspect of human existence. The emergence of HIV has made prison sexuality a public health issue[4]. Here, the questioning stems first and foremost from a reflection on the redefinition of the objectives of deprivation of liberty. Several centuries ago, Cesare Beccaria wrote that, to achieve its objective, a punishment must be *just, proportionate* and *defined*[5]. In light of our contemporary society and fundamental human rights, is France's current prison system capable of meeting these three conditions? What's at stake is its credibility and effectiveness in adapting to what people's consciences are no longer ashamed to name. That's why, behind the prism of sexuality, this sociological approach feeds a critical vision of the penal institution, its intrinsic limits and the danger it represents in a democratic society.

Human sexuality remains a mystery that is becoming better understood by the day. The prison population recognizes it as the direct or indirect causal origin of the majority of offences committed. Psychoanalysis sees it as the driving force behind desires and the underpinning of life drives. *Lifting the veil* on sexual practices in the prison environment, and at the same time attempting to put into words the expectations of inmates, supervisory staff, management and medical staff, constitutes a sociological challenge in the context of the secrecy of penitentiary alcoves, making taboos talkable at last. The deprivation of pleasure, the narrowing of the senses, the subjection of an intrinsically human practice to authorization or prohibition in the context of deprivation of

---

4. LHUILIER (Dominique), RIDEL (Luc), SIMONPIETRI (Aldona), VEIL (Claude), *Identité professionnelle, identité de sexe et sida : le cas des surveillants de prison*, Université Paris VII, Laboratoire de psychologie clinique, March 1998, p. 101.
5. BECCARIA (Cesare), *Des délits et des peines*, Paris, Flammarion, 1991.

liberty, necessarily has a meaning, an origin, the roots of which cannot be conceived independently of the difficulties we are experiencing today in dealing with this issue. Difficulties in thinking, in dialogue, in exposing this reflection, and the concrete implementation that should result from it, to the public arena. Above all, we're finding it hard to reach a consensus, to turn this issue into a matter of course. Perhaps tomorrow it will become unbearable to think that prisons could have been conceived without authorized, organized sexual practices?

As with Goffman's conclusions, the analysis of a total institution highlights functions and behaviours that are as many objectifiable variables whose scope governs our society in a more general way. More often than not, prisons are viewed only by the individuals who make them up: the inmate population on the one hand, prison administration staff on the other, but also by a series of more or less independent players, ranging from healthcare professionals to justice professionals, not forgetting education, training and the voluntary sector. All have a vision of the institution based on daily immersion, through which the meaning of things is first justified before being analyzed. The interest of sociological work in prisons lies in the willingness to insert an outside, independent observer into a social reality from which he or she is not fundamentally excluded, but which for him or her constitutes neither an authority issue nor a means of legitimization. On the one hand, this difference in viewpoint has motivated the authorizations for access granted by school managements, and on the other, has led to numerous refusals, on the grounds that knowledge constitutes power and therefore a risk likely to shake an inertia that is sometimes skilfully nurtured.

This study brings together two objects whose respective interests are particularly opposed. And therein lies the challenge: prison is often perceived as a forgotten object, devoid of interest, dark and depressing, while the mere mention of the word *sexuality* arouses an interest that is as manifest as it is frequent. Finally, the combination of this work, placing interest in the contingency of disinterest, opens up unexpected horizons of curiosity, stemming from a mixture of the *taboo* and the *intimate*. On the borders of psychological and psychoanalytical dimensions, the aim here is to contrast the *living together* required by resocialization, with the destructuring of the relationship to oneself and the relationship to otherness, analyzed as consequences of incarceration in long sentences[6]. It is with this hypothesis in mind that this paper examines the place of sexuality in the sentencing mechanism, with regard to rehabilitation objectives.

The economies of power that are woven in detention around sexual issues are also played out within the prison population, in the elaboration of human relationships and the social bonds that make up prison society. Sexuality generates relationships of interest, identification and implicit contracts, the aim of which is to satisfy frustrated desires and altered identity images. In prison, sexuality stigmatizes individuals from an intimacy deviated to the collective, to the point of producing a social hierarchy elaborated according to a scale of values that redefines, within detention, the contours of good and evil, the acceptable and the punishable, respectable humanity and definitively degraded beings.

---

6. The definition of *long sentences* is relative. Given that the vast majority of short sentences do not exceed six or eight months, *long sentences* frequently refer to sentences of two years or more. This work focuses on the discourse of a population detained for more than 5 years.

PART ONE

PRISONS AND INMATES

Prologue
Who are they?
Individual prisoner stories

Among the male and female prisoners we met, here is a presentation of those whose words particularly inspired this analysis. To ensure confidentiality, each interviewee was asked to identify himself using a pseudonym of his choice.

- Saturnin is 39 years old. He is incarcerated at the Œrmingen detention center after being sentenced to eight years for raping an under-age girl. He has already served four years, and hopes to be released in two years. Saturnin is married with two children. He was a truck driver. With incarceration, he declares that today, his libido is down to zero: "I never think about it, I don't get an erection in the morning, sometimes during the night, it surprises me and I laugh looking at my sex."

- Zizou is 28 years old. He is incarcerated at the Saint-Mihiel detention center for seven years, convicted of drug trafficking. He is single and considers that he became a *man when*, at the age of 16, he had his first sexual encounter, thanks to a sensual trap organized by his older brother. By not practicing, he's "afraid I won't be able to perform anymore, that I won't know how to practice". "I'm able to channel my fears and compensate with sport. During a leave, he met a young girl with whom he had sexual relations, uninhibited by alcohol to give himself confidence.

- Myriam is 25 years old. She is incarcerated at the Bapaume detention center, having been sentenced to eighteen years for "theft with violence resulting in death without intent". Myriam was previously incarcerated at the Rennes women's detention center. There, she benefited from the experimentation of Family Visiting Units (UVF)[7]. On the first occasion with her boyfriend, she admits that she was particularly keen to have sex. The other times, she received her immediate family.

- Marseille is 34 years old. She is incarcerated at the Bapaume detention center, having been convicted over eighteen years ago of murdering the legionnaire who had raped her best friend. Marseille develops violent outbursts that she frequently turns against herself. In this case, at the time of the interview, she had two recent stab wounds on her neck, which she tries to hide with a scarf during visits to the visiting room. When she was incarcerated, her son had just been born. And every week since then, her son, now 18, and his partner have flown in from Corsica for a few hours of visiting time. Marseille has already been granted leave on several occasions. She has thus been able to resume her life on the outside, and in these decent conditions, has been able to resume a sexual and love life with her husband.

- Mulder is 45 years old. He has been detained in Saint-Mihiel for six years after being convicted of sexually assaulting a 15-year-old boy. According to him, the charge stemmed from revenge on the part of his

---

7. Family Visiting Units (UVF) are still the exception, where prisoners can meet their loved ones for up to 72 hours. This is the French adaptation of the "parloirs sexuels", which allow conjugal encounters.

ex-wife. Mulder has one child, whom he has not seen since his incarceration. Mulder has always loved women and men equally. In prison, he is friends with three other sex offenders or homosexuals, with whom he has established sufficient complicity not to have to suffer too much from the ostracism that the whole of detention subjects him to.

- Armand is 66 years old. He is incarcerated at the Val-de-Reuil detention center for an eighteen-year prison sentence for the rape of two under-age boys, for which he served nine years. His wife has remained faithful to him and visits him several times a year in the visiting room. During his childhood, and while his father was stationed abroad, Armand remembers being raped. His mother always denied this. He evokes a comparative vision between the army and prison, while noting a notable difference in matters of sexuality. In his day, the French state, through the army, recognized individual sexual needs and provided prostitutes for all garrisons based abroad.

- Lucien is 61 years old. He is incarcerated at the Val-de-Reuil detention center for having had sexual relations with underage girls for many years: "In all, I had a maximum of ten girls, I did it with entire families, the eldest passing on the baton to the youngest." Lucien was a marble mason, working with the gravediggers. He is divorced, with three children. His life was turned upside down when, at a young age, he was diagnosed with intestinal cancer. Since then, he has survived thanks to an artificial anus. From then on, he felt diminished, his wife refused to have intimate relations with him, and he turned to very young girls. At the age of 10, Lucien was raped by the dentist at a summer camp. Prior to the interview, he had never spoken of this event again, except to the psychiatrist treating him in detention. Lucien has been sentenced to life imprisonment. He has already spent sixteen years in prison, and hopes to be released in four years.

- Ryan, aged 20, is a multi-recidivist prisoner sentenced this time to twenty months at the Saint-Mihiel detention center. Ryan does not meet the criteria for long sentences as defined in this study. However, the fact that he had already spent several years in prison, in several different sentences, and above all, that he himself had requested to take part in the interview, motivated the acceptance of his testimony. Ryan feels that society is not suited to him. He needs extreme moments that cost sums he's not prepared to earn at the sacrifice of a youth that calls him to multiple pleasures. As a result, he confided that he would continue to return regularly to "square prison" out of a refusal to conform to the social norm. Incarceration is seen as an incidental risk, and has no credibility for him.

- Marcus is 39 years old. He was convicted of murder and sentenced to twenty years' imprisonment, with a thirteen-year security period. Marcus has long traded in his charms, through prostitution, erotic shows and *X-rated films*. He claims to have been bisexual since childhood, although the homosexuality he practiced was often motivated by professional and financial reasons. Marcus was sexually abused as a child by both men and women. In the end, it was because he killed a *pointer*[8] that he now finds himself in prison. Marcus is Austrian. Like most inmates of foreign nationality, he will not be granted leave or parole in France, regardless of his behavior. The prison administration is afraid of escapes to his country of origin. On the other hand, he knows that, on his return to Austria, he will benefit from a reintegration process that will guarantee him a job and accommodation on his release. Mainly as a drug user, he has been incarcerated in Germany, Austria, Italy, Greece and France.

---

8. The word *pointeur* belongs to prison jargon. It's a synonym for *rapist*. Initially, it referred more to adult rapists. Today, with the emphasis on the repression of paedophilia, *pointers* also, and almost primarily, refer to child rapists.

- Léon is 29 years old. He is incarcerated in Val-de-Reuil for murder. He was sexually molested when he was 8, by his uncle and his neighbor. Now, he says of the pointers: "I have a deep-seated hatred of paedophiles, and I wonder if I'm the one who turned them on. In fact, the simple act of scratching one's genitals... they took it as teasing!" On the other hand, his sexual appetite makes him accept any proposition, as long as it involves a woman. He has already had a sexual relationship in detention with a female guard, taking care to specify that it was "in another detention center". Because his partners recognize that they are unable to satisfy his sexual needs, they accept that he has relations outside the couple. Given the sexual needs he expresses, the ban on sexual relations is a source of great suffering for him.

- Jason is 28 years old. He was convicted of murder and sentenced to fifteen years' imprisonment. He has already served eight years and hopes to be released in five. Jason has a child, and rather than live out his marital relationship in the destitution that incarceration allows, he preferred to break up, and move geographically away from his partner to be closer to his son (whom he had previously had with another woman). Jason explained that his girlfriend was very curious about how inmates might experience their sexuality in prison. She seemed very excited by the prohibition to be defied.

- Tony is 32 years old. He is incarcerated at the Saint-Mihiel detention center. He was sentenced to eight years for armed robbery, of which he served the first four. Tony claims to be a seducer, and in fact appears to be flirtatious and concerned about his physical appearance and the size of his muscles. He also presents himself as a "jouisseur", a gourmand of life's pleasures, between food, drink and women, he admits to having great needs.

- Tom is 37 years old. He is incarcerated at the Œrmingen detention center. He has been sentenced to fifteen years for murdering his wife's lover. Tom doesn't always have a job in prison. He is also involved in a choir and chaplaincy. He acknowledges that some people don't have sex outside prison either, often out of religious choice, but that inside prison, the fact that the ban is subjectively experienced as a constraint gives rise to manifestations of violence and aggression.

- Françoise is 48 years old. She is incarcerated at the Bapaume detention center, convicted of failing to denounce the sexual abuse her husband committed against several of their children (boys and girls). Françoise has five children. She confides that sexuality has always been a compulsory practice to which she has submitted under social or cultural constraint, which positions women as objects for the satisfaction of the husband's desire, and the female body as a means of reproduction. Françoise has never masturbated, and doesn't know the meaning of any of the terms, practices or notions mentioned. She explains that sexuality is completely foreign to her, and as such, prison frees her from daily sexual obligations.

- Stéphane is 39 years old. He was sentenced to twenty-two years' imprisonment in Val-de-Reuil for a crime of passion. The separation from his wife plunged him into a deep depression. A double murder followed. Stéphane has already spent eleven years in prison. He expects to be released soon. Sexuality, as a practice independent of feelings, is not essential for Stéphane. In fact, his attention to women and the satisfaction of desire has disappeared since his incarceration. It's now that his release is imminent that he's starting to think about women again: "Now, with the idea of parole looming, I've been asking myself this question of pleasing again for about two years. I'm trying to get interested in other women, I'm starting to look at them again. There are times when it's hard. You think about it, but it's never a priority."

- Garouda is 59 years old. He is incarcerated at the Caen detention center, having been sentenced to fifteen years' imprisonment for *incesting* his daughter. He was an electrician in the navy, which enabled him to travel a lot, and to experiment sexually with prostituted women, military men like himself, and sometimes even animals. At the age of 17, he was raped by a military doctor, then by a legionnaire. Garouda has great sexual needs, and because he realizes the growing importance of sexual delinquency, he is very interested in the therapies developed in Canada and in alternative sentences to combat recidivism. He alternates between men and women. While in prison, he has several lovers, with whom he engages in homosexual practices as both penetrator and penetrated. This does not exclude his desire for a woman, which he fulfils on his release.

- Saul is 24 years old. He is incarcerated at the Saint-Mihiel detention center. He is Brazilian; his father, who stays in regular contact with him from Brazil, is an Adventist pastor. Saul's recent conversion has given him a more optimistic outlook on his future. Today, however, he struggles to reconcile religious precepts with the substitute sexuality he is forced to indulge in prison to appease his libido. Saul was sentenced to twelve years' imprisonment for a murder he committed in French Guiana. He has already served five years in prison, and expects to be released in four years.

- Damien is 42 years old. He is held at the Val-de-Reuil detention center. He was convicted as a multi-recidivist for rape of a minor and murder. His case was widely publicized in the 1990s. He was sentenced to life imprisonment, with a twenty-five year security sentence. Damien says he was never integrated into society. His youth alternated between boarding schools, placements at the DDASS, incarceration and periods of vagrancy. Around the age of 14, he was abused by an educator. Today, he admits to being wary of "slightly affectionate" adults. Damien admits to being a compulsive paedophile. The prison governor explains that during a recent search, a notebook filled with photos of children cut out from mail-order catalogs was discovered in his cell. This practice is common in detention, for paedophiles who have no means of acquiring illegal paedophile erotica.

- Franck, 37, was sentenced to fifteen years' imprisonment for sexual offences against under-age boys. He is being held in Val-de-Reuil. He was raped at the age of 8 by one of his older brothers, with whom he continued an incestuous relationship for a long time. Franck also tried zoophilia when he was 12. He loves both men and women. His intense sexual need was often satisfied by furtive relationships that he accumulated during the day, as a sexual complement to his heterosexual couple relationship. Today, he is divorced with a child he no longer sees. Franck has 5 years' higher education and used to work for Renault. In prison, he is sociable and respected by everyone. His tolerant attitude and personality mean that he doesn't suffer from the anathema heaped on pointers and homosexuals. He's been through the worst, and the worst is what he's done and the consequences: confinement, distance from his son, social hatred and self-contempt. Nothing and nobody scares him anymore.

- Bruce is 38 years old. He is incarcerated for the first time at the Val-de-Reuil detention center, for voluntary manslaughter. He was sentenced to fifteen years' imprisonment. To date, he has served six, and expects to be out in three or four years. For him, sexuality and prison are incompatible. At the age of 14, Bruce was raped by five men, all of whom are now serving prison sentences. He still has nightmares about it. Bruce has a son, and explains that he suffers a lot from loneliness. The solution for him would be to be able to meet his son more frequently and for longer. In addition, Bruce suffers from a series of pathologies that make him increasingly disabled (80% disability: genetic disease, arteritis/arthrosis, cardiovascular accident). He walks with a crutch and has to take powerful painkillers.

- Doudou is 43 years old. He is incarcerated in Val-de-Reuil. He was sentenced to twenty years for murdering a minor. He has been locked up for eleven years and expects to be released in two years. Doudou was successively an EDF agent and a professional gambler (racing, poker, etc.). He confessed to having long had problems with alcohol, which he tried to cure in numerous rehabs. In the end, being in detention enabled him to make a complete withdrawal. In exchange, Doudou is prescribed anxiolytics, sleeping pills and antidepressants, which he uses in his own way. Every week, he overdoses on Atimil, swallowing the seven-day dosage in one go: "That way, I get rid of a day in prison every week."

- Bruno is 40 years old. He is being held at the Val-de-Reuil prison, having been sentenced to twelve years' imprisonment for having sexual relations with a boy under the age of 15. After obtaining a master's degree in maritime law, Bruno worked in New Caledonia as a specialized educator in an open environment, for the justice system and the DDASS. He found New Caledonian teenagers to be younger and more mature than their counterparts in mainland France, with a particular sexual freedom. He doesn't feel that he raped his lover. However, the age difference between the two partners was the reason for a relationship he felt was inappropriate. That's why Bruno chose to turn himself in to the local authorities. A few months later, this relationship would not have been punishable.

- Fabrice is 42 years old. He is serving a ten-year prison sentence at the Val-de-Reuil detention center. He was convicted of having a sexual relationship with a 13-year-old girl. He states that there was no coercion or penetration. Given the age of his partner, the sexual act is considered rape, and Fabrice is considered a punching bag within the detention center. In his youth, Fabrice was sexually abused: "I was raped when I was 7 by an adult (someone from the village), a notable person, so it never came to light. The fact that I talked about it at the time, and yet it was never acknowledged, raises problems of guilt and forgetting. In fact, this story came back to me through the therapy I underwent in prison."

- Charles is 54 years old. He is serving a life sentence at the Val-de-Reuil detention center, for voluntary manslaughter. He has already spent twenty-four years in prison, and expects to be released soon with a spouse, a teacher he met in prison. Charles trained as an anthropologist. He regularly publishes articles on society and politics. He has no hatred of sex offenders: "I try to understand, I have no positive or negative judgments. I try to be neutral, to assume the aftermath and I look for the usefulness of prison for them... They have nothing to do in prison, it would be better to have other structures."

- Prof is 27 years old and has been incarcerated in Œrmingen for three years as a multi-recidivist drug dealer. Prof has very moral conceptions of right and wrong, which he claims are rooted in his Muslim upbringing. He associates paedophilia and homosexuality in a register of deviances that should be punished by death: "They're all paedophiles (homosexuals), I'd cut my son's head off if he told me he was gay!" On the subject of substitute homosexuality in detention, he says: "I'd rather hang myself than let myself fall into the pleasures of life [*sic*], even if I'm in for life."

- Sly is 46 years old. He is incarcerated in Œrmingen. He has been living with his current partner for twenty-two years. He has had no children with her, but has raised the three daughters she already had. It was this decisive fact that enabled his partner to forgive him for the acts

Sly committed against two of her daughters. During the investigation, Sly spent two years at liberty. Then he was incarcerated for five years, of which he hopes to serve only half. His conviction is socially too shameful to be made official. As head of a cleaning company, knowledge of this offence would scare off all the customers. So his concubine has to pretend he's away on business or training, to justify his disappearance. Sly sees the consequences of his imprisonment in the social and financial decline he suffers following his incarceration. He finds it all the more difficult to come to terms with his sentence, given that the facts date back nineteen years, and that after the fact, he considers himself to have behaved like a "good family man", enabling his three adopted daughters to build up an enviable social and family life.

- Wolf is 56 years old. He is a German national. He was sentenced to life imprisonment for a series of robberies, a murder and an escape. He spent twenty-one years in prison, both in Germany and France. Wolf benefited from a new French law which allows release in cases of incurable illness[9]. He has been operated on several times for cancer on his face. Since then, so as not to force him back into detention, the doctors outside refuse to sign a certificate attesting that he is cured. In fact, Wolf was met in Paris on his way to receive comfort care following the treatments he had undergone. For him, the greatest disruption caused by imprisonment is the break-up of his family.

- Hervé is 51 years old and has been incarcerated at the Caen detention center for 27 years for a homicide he now admits he committed because he didn't accept his homosexuality. At the time, he needed to "sadize" the men with whom he shared the beginnings of sexual relations. He even went so far as to kill. In prison, he runs the video workshop that

---

9. Law of March 4, 2002.

feeds an internal channel, with programs in which he welcomes guests, some of them renowned, to talk about prison conditions in particular.

- Oiseau Rouge is 45 years old. She is an elegant, smiling, flirtatious woman. She is of French nationality and African descent. As such, her upbringing does not encourage her to verbalize her sexuality. All the more so since Oiseau Rouge declares herself to be very religious: "I pray in my cell and listen to a church song every morning." She is incarcerated at the Bapaume detention center, where she has been serving a 30-year sentence for twelve years, for a crime of passion. She is alleged to have encouraged the drowning of one of her husband's mistresses. Oiseau Rouge suffers from a lack of freedom, and submission to the conditions of confinement is added to her previous submission to her ex-spouse, to the point that even though she now declares that she is in love, she refuses the idea of a marriage that would lock her up again. Oiseau Rouge also suffers from a lack of sexuality, tenderness and pleasure. Her libido is said to be reduced to nothing, and the absence of sexual relations has, according to her doctor, caused physiological dysfunctions in her ovaries. Oiseau Rouge has a 20-year-old daughter. On the outside, she worked as a cleaner for the Ministry of Education. Inside, she helps a fellow inmate look after her baby.

- Nanou is 54 years old. She is incarcerated at the Bapaume detention center for killing her grandson's rapist. Like many incarcerated women, Nanou has lived a life of violence and domination. In the end, she took refuge in alcohol. She herself had previously been raped several times, then beaten and possessed by a jealous and overbearing husband, sometimes to the point of hospitalization after he had, for example, decided to run her over with his car. Finally, it was at the Bapaume detention center that Nanou realized that the platonic lover of her adolescence was himself incarcerated in the men's section of the same establishment. They began writing letters and exchanging photos, and Nanou is now thinking of marrying the man who brings her love and comfort during their weekly meetings in the visiting room. When she says, with regard to prostitution, that women are neither interested nor strategic, she is also referring to her own situation. Indeed, the courts were prepared to be particularly lenient in the face of her crime of defense, until, motivated by sentiment, she rushed her request for permission to marry her newfound lover, incarcerated for acts of pedophilia. In the end, falling in love with a paedophile while trying to justify why she had murdered another paedophile led to a particularly long sentence.

- Geronimo is 34 years old. He has been imprisoned at the Val-de-Reuil detention center for six years, for committing a murder for which he was sentenced to twenty-five years' imprisonment. His release is scheduled for 2015. Geronimo had already spent eight years in prison. Between these two incarcerations, he worked as a gardener in an amusement park. After being sexually abused between the ages of 13 and 16, Geronimo was raped by fellow inmates at the prison for over a month. The warden did not want to publicize the case, so the offence went unpunished. Two years ago, he got married on prison premises, to the mother of one of his friends. He points out that sexuality is not essential to him. In fact, between his long years of incarceration and his relative lack of libido, Geronimo admits to having had only twenty or so sexual encounters in his entire life.

- Augustin is 21 years old. He is incarcerated in Saint-Mihiel for theft with violence against the police. Augustin has already spent five years in prison, with several convictions. He describes himself as bisexual. He hopes to be released in twenty-one months. He had already been sentenced eight times as a juvenile for similar offences. Augustin doesn't like working, but enjoys a relatively high standard of living. As a result, he has been a regular prostitute since the age of 9: "A 40-year-old man lured me with a 500-franc bill. I didn't realize it. I knew it wasn't right, but as long as nobody knew, it didn't bother me. Today, I regret it. It was an ongoing relationship, but he was using me." Augustin adds: "It's not the job that motivates me, it's the money you make. I almost became a boner because it pays 3,000 euros a month, but in fact, it disgusts me too much." Augustin had previously discovered sexuality with a 36-year-old woman when he was 7 or 8. He never wanted to make the sexual violence he experienced official, for fear of triggering new bouts of violence in his father. So he waited until after his father's death to start talking to psychologists. Augustin, who feels aroused by all women in general, points out that the lack of sexual relations makes inmates perverse. Prison, he says, causes sexual instability, and in the end the women who agree to meet prisoners in need know very well "what they want to find there".

- Francis is 48 years old. He has been incarcerated for twenty-two years for homicide. He is currently serving the remainder of his sentence at the Caen detention center, where he has met his new partner (a pointer and heterosexual before his incarceration), with whom he has just entered into a civil union. The latter, who was released prematurely, has just taken an apartment next to the prison, in order to have easier access to the visiting rooms. In the 1970s, Francis spent a brief period in show business as a singer. He still has some contacts with this profession, which is enough to nourish a few illusions as to the possible rebirth, after liberation, of a career that never really got off the ground.

- Dany, 42, is incarcerated at the Bapaume detention center for covering up a crime committed by her partner. According to her, her silence was motivated by blackmail and threats of violence against herself and her children. Dany is now in a relationship with another inmate, younger than herself, with whom she shares a cell. She knows that her partner is unfaithful, and blames her for it, but admits that she is not sexually satisfied, especially as her sexual needs are increasingly focused on the need for daily tenderness and the need not to sleep without snuggling up to a loving body. Dany has four children. Her eldest daughter was recently raped four times, by men who have just been sentenced to ten years' imprisonment. She herself discovered sexuality when she was raped at the age of 4 by her stepfather, who was never convicted. She subsequently suffered further rapes and violence at the hands of authoritarian, domineering spouses. Today, Dany doesn't stop herself from being seduced by men as a virile image, but has no desire to ever unite with a man again, given her traumatic memories.

- Serge, 50, is incarcerated at the Val-de-Reuil detention center, following a conviction for armed robbery. This is now the sixth year he has served for this offence, for which he was sentenced to fourteen years. Given his generation and delinquent background, Serge is the "prototypical bank robber". He had five previous convictions for the same offence, including a nineteen-year sentence. In the end, Serge spent half his life in prison. Between the two main incarcerations, he redeemed his conduct by "making deals". "The cops liked it and thought I was tidy," he says, but with a spending pattern more in keeping with the purchasing power of a bank robber than a shopkeeper, Serge had to hang up his life of crime to pay off debts. "Bank robbery was all I really knew how to do. In my generation, you don't take from the little guys, so you have to go and get the dough where it's at." Serge was betrayed by the driver he had hired. "I took on a driver who didn't belong to the business, so as not to be *rehired*. He got arrested for drunkenness one day, and as he wasn't a member of organized crime, he went straight to the table." Serge has two children. He says he's always been a "hothead", with a lot of "experience to make up for" between incarcerations. A self-confessed infidel, he claims to have always had a companion during his periods of incarceration. His sexual practices in the visiting room are limited to caresses. He doesn't want to try any further out of respect for women.

- Henry is 32 years old. He is serving his prison sentence at the Saint-Mihiel detention center. He was sentenced to seven years for murder. He considers that he acted in self-defense. He has already spent five years in prison and hopes to be released in a few months. Henry believes that prison would become too comfortable if conjugal sex were allowed. He has known inmates in prison who, on the day of their release, would say to him: "Keep my bed, I'll be back soon, I'm better off in prison than out!" He doesn't see any particular lack of sexuality and doesn't intend to have a sexual relationship without an emotional investment that doesn't fit in with the circumstances of confinement.

- Xavier is 48 years old. He is incarcerated at the Val-de-Reuil detention center, for murdering the man who wanted to prostitute his daughter in Holland. He was sentenced to twenty-five years. After serving eleven years, he will be released on parole. Xavier was the owner of a well-known restaurant in a provincial town. Due to the quality of its services, his establishment was the region's preferred venue for the "local elite". High-ranking gendarmerie officials rubbed shoulders with the local mafia, and when Xavier realized the intentions of the pimping clients with regard to his own daughter, he tried to obtain special protection for her: "They [the gendarmes] were complicit with the bandits, and wouldn't take into account what I was asking of them. During the trial, they even advised me to keep quiet about the dirty cops...". Distraught at the prospect of his daughter being sent to Holland to be prostituted in a shop window, and faced with a refusal to cooperate on the part of the gendarmerie, Xavier took the risk of defending his offspring himself. He killed the two criminals. This story has a great deal of credibility within the prison system. In fact, Xavier is a man who is highly respected by the prison population, including all prison staff. His gesture is understood by all, making him a kind of *heroic father with a big heart.*

- Max is 34 years old. He is incarcerated at the Œrmingen detention center for violence and fighting. This time, he has been sentenced to thirty months. In this sense, he does not meet the criteria for long sentences, except that as a multi-recidivist, he has spent more than seven years in prison over the last twelve years. Max has been living with the same woman for thirteen years. By now, he and his partner have become accustomed to allowing their sexuality to survive regardless of prison restrictions. "This time," he says, "she warned me that this is the last time she'll put up with my delinquent acts. She's really been very patient, and I'd like to stay out longer so we can build good memories."

- Alfred is 64 years old and has been incarcerated at the Œrmingen detention center for five years. He was sentenced to fifteen years for raping a 15-year-old girl. He expects to be released in four years. Alfred started out as a miner, then enrolled at the Technical College. After an accident in the mines, he attended gendarmerie school. Following marital difficulties, he left the civil service. He went to work in a German foundry to support his family. At the age of 30, doctors diagnosed him with multiple sclerosis. He became an invalid, paralyzed for a time. He began rehabilitation, walking again with two canes, and claims that his remission is due to a fierce will to survive: "I threw away the second cane a little while ago." Alfred recently took part in a poetry competition organized by the department. Ironically, he won first prize with a poem ambiguously describing the sensual affection between a man and children. The detention center's psychiatrist explained that he had explained to the warden that such an *adventure* was probably not the best idea for a pedophile.

Chapter 1
Sexuality behind the walls

Numerous definitions, whether philosophical, sociological, psychological, physiological, literary, cultural or historical, force us to delimit, if not limit, what we mean by human sexuality. We have adopted a deliberately broad conception of sexuality as a global notion, touching on the physical, psychic and social existence of individuals. Sexuality is recognition, limits, good and evil, pleasure and pain, life and death, liaison and relationship, carnal and affective, virtual or real, what Louis-Ferdinand Céline defined as "the most subtle in man". It is undoubtedly this part of the *living being* that oscillates between the singular and the collective, between intimacy and sharing, between the bodily senses and the investment of the soul, between selfless giving and the search for identity. It represents a book, sometimes open, sometimes closed, in which individual narratives are copiously recorded. To speak of sexuality is often to evoke only the existence and use of the so-called "sexual" organs. But because lived experience is not limited to acts, evoking sexuality means exploring a territory with unknown frontiers and experiences as numerous as the singularity of the intimacies questioned.

In addition to the urinary functions of the penis and vagina, sex is the organ of reproduction, of the life we come from and the life we give. It's also the word most languages use to describe one's gender. Finally, it's the word that designates the place of physical pleasure, for which we too easily forget the collaboration of other senses, which involve considering the physical body as a whole, including those thoughts immaterialized in the brain tissue.

With the avowed aim of approaching a global analysis of the sentencing mechanism, it is also the implications of the sexual dimension in existences that need to be interpreted here on the basis of typologies defined by sexual behaviors, orientations, types of practices, and the diversity of needs that this fieldwork has enabled us to typologize. This enables us to understand social mechanisms at the heart of an institution which, within its walls, reconstitutes a society in its own right, in which the interests of individual survival always take the place of the general interest.

The official regime of sexuality in French prisons

> "It is a second-degree disciplinary offence for a prisoner to: [...]
> 5° - Perform obscene acts or acts likely to offend public decency;
> [...]".[10]

It's as if prison, in its original conception, had omitted the question of sexuality. Article D. 249-2 paragraph 5 of the Code of Criminal Procedure is the legal basis for the regime imposed on sexuality in the prison environment. There is in fact no prohibition in principle, other than the fact that the configuration of detention facilities does not allow sexual practices to be carried out away from prying eyes or involuntary views, likely to offend the modesty of warders, other inmates, families and even children present in the visiting room. It's not so much a question

---

10. Article D. 249-2 paragraph 5 of the Code of Criminal Procedure.

of a formal prohibition on sexual relations, as of a prohibition discreetly concealed behind contempt for a need, which both architecture and jurists have endeavored to forget. The legal argument underpinning the fate of some 60,000 prisoners[11] is performative, yet paradoxically completely silent on the object it describes. The imperceptible mention of sexuality behind the allusions to *obscenity* and *modesty* generates such consequences for prisoners that we can't help but wonder about the disproportion between a ban that is so poorly motivated on the one hand, and consequences that are so heavily suffered on the other. In spite of this de facto ban, it seems that nature and needs express themselves regularly. *Baby visiting rooms* exist, and stories of sexual relations more or less made possible are legion. Whether voluntary or involuntary, these pregnancies represent a negation of prison life in all its prohibitions and deprivations. The prospect of this new life to come contrasts with the restrictive horizon of monosexual confinement.

It's finally accepted that a *wrongdoer* remains a *wrongdoer*, that wrong-doing deserves punishment, and that the effectiveness of punishment is proportional to the intensity of the constraint exerted. Prison is vengeance for some and coercion for others. In both cases, it represents the power of order, obedience, control and the forms of submission established as the foundation of an organized society that seeks to reassure the integrity of property, people and institutions. Franck, incarcerated in Val-de-Reuil, explains without illusion: "Society doesn't want us to be good, it wants us to be nothing." Controlling sexuality comes into play in this perspective, by emphasizing to offenders that the temporary suspension of their adult autonomy is made necessary by the sense of danger posed to others by delinquent behavior. Paradoxically, it is by depriving inmates of a share of otherness, particularly in the

---

11. The number of inmates has hovered around 60,000 for several years. On April 1st, 2008, a record 63,120 people were in prison.

sexual dimension, that prison intends to act as a deterrent before being a redemptive solution.

Desire or dematerialized sexuality

Beyond practices, sexuality is understood here first and foremost as a desire, analyzable as the conscious or unconscious feeling of a need for the other as an object of excitation and as a *fellow being* to be encountered. The other can be understood as a metaphor for a part of oneself, according to the Platonic definition of the episode in which the anger of the gods led to the splitting of the human being "as one cuts an egg with a hair"[12]. Similarly, the authority of judges in society leads to the separation of lovers. Plato explains that, as a result of this wrath, "regretting his half", each aspires to find it again, to embrace it, "with the desire to melt together". Fabienne Casta-Rosaz analyzes this story as one of the definitions of sexuality, justifying the extent to which this intrinsic desire, common to a large proportion of living beings, takes on a very special dimension when it comes to human beings[13].

Sexuality as understood by prisoners, in a place where practices are either prohibited or made difficult by the very conditions of incarceration, is expressed first and foremost as a *desire to*. Excitement born of an image, an encounter, a smell, a memory, constitutes a form of sexuality, sometimes residual when nothing else is feasible. Even if one prisoner confessed: "In prison, I'm a nun", fantasy activity, because of the split between desire and its fulfillment, is the sexuality most frequently experienced by prisoners. In the manner of Descartes' "I think, therefore I am", the observation goes something like this: "I enjoy, therefore

---

12. PLATO, *Le Banquet*, Paris, Flammarion, 1998, p. 115.
13. CASTA-ROSAZ (Fabienne), *Histoire de la sexualité en Occident*, Paris, La Martinière, 2004, p. 7.

there's always happiness to be had in the present; even in prison I get hard, therefore I'm still a man."[14] Whether contemporary or past, this study relies on discourses as performatives of a reality that makes or has made sense, in the interviewees' journey. When a prisoner confides: "The libido disappears in prison", this absence of confessed sexuality constitutes in itself a form of sexuality, disappeared of course, but nonetheless the object of analysis.

Sexuality defined by the senses

When asked: "Where do you think sexuality begins?", the answer invariably refers to organs other than the pubic area. It's usually a look, a touch, a smell. Sexuality begins with desire, through the stimulation of the senses, even before it becomes a behavioral practice. As Sigmund Freud concluded, the use of the genitals is *just one* of the achievements of sexuality[15].

To express the *beginning of the sexual,* the male inmates speak of "looking", of simply "thinking about it", while the women speak of an "attraction" that must be "shared and reciprocated". The men seem to have this need to combine their singularity with a woman whose subjectively apprehended qualities are so many parameters in the construction of the evaluation with their fellow men. Women, on the other hand, adopt a more pragmatic attitude, aiming to satisfy a desire of their own, disregarding the added value that the object of desire brings to their evaluation within the female gender community. This is how Myriam, an inmate at Bapaume, expresses her approach to sexuality: "For me

---

14. MARCHETTI (Anne-Marie), *Perpétuités. Le temps infini des longues peines*, Paris, Plon, coll. "Terre humaine", 2001, p. 233.
15. FREUD (Sigmund), *Abrégé de psychanalyse*, Paris, PUF, coll. "Bibliothèque de psychanalyse", 1975, p. 13.

to sleep with a woman here, I'd already have to find an attractive one. I'm not attracted to any of them; they're all old, ugly and deformed." Marseille adds: "Sexuality begins with words, which have no sexual connotations in terms of satisfying the senses. It's simply an invitation to have a drink, to eat in a restaurant, anything that creates a kind of attraction and trust."

When men exist as a function of competition within their own gender, women enjoy greater detachment. When men's violence is instrumentalized to assert a valuation of power, women become more obsessed with satisfying the singularity of their desires, and organizing the durability of their satisfaction.

In the prisoners' discourse, sexuality appears first and foremost as the encounter between two desires, which are expressed or recognized by sight, hearing, smell or touch. Sexuality begins with a desire to show tenderness to someone we meet, as well as to receive it. Disregarding the views of some male inmates, who may express the desire to penetrate and *discharge* as an exclusive need, the definition of sexuality is adorned with the trappings of affect, contemplation, and the birth of a reassuring reciprocity, in which an intimate game between two people is established.

Sexuality is also defined by opportunities of time and space. Discotheques are frequently cited as a kind of agora, staging a market of supply and demand. It is also this *place of all possibilities* that is lacking in prison. From the very beginnings of relationships that men describe as sexual, a power struggle is woven, whose ambiguity is instrumentalized for the benefit of growing excitement. Ambiguity is one of the abstractions that define sexuality, based on a random feeling of possession of the other, or of giving oneself to the other. Sexual practice constitutes this alchemy between the concreteness of bodies, the mechanics of organs and a whole series of spiritual and sensory abstractions that posit the present moment as the certainty of being alive, a certainty ultimately as irrational and precarious as the very idea of death.

The point of these definitions was to understand the place of otherness in the sexuality thus described. The conclusions were quickly organized around the notions of *missing otherness* in solitary sexuality, *forbidden otherness in the* context of homosexuality, or *controlled* otherness in conjugal encounters in the visiting room. The sexuality of which prisoners are deprived in detention is presented as sharing, a practice that is gradually learned and that enables the discovery of *the other self* through the exchange of satisfactions and the stakes of success that ensue. Saturnin speaks of "mutual exchange, because [he] likes to please", suggesting a reciprocity as much in desire and need, as in satisfaction. Zizou speaks of "looks and gestures, and a whole lot of things that don't deceive", and thus confers on conjugated sexuality the parameter of obviousness that is lacking behind the walls.

The *rupture* between outside and inside practices

The major problem of sexuality in the prison environment begins with the *disruptive effect of* imprisonment. Each person was asked about his or her sexual history, starting with the discovery of pleasure, either alone or with one or more partners. They were also asked to talk about their sexuality, based on their perception of their couple or extra-marital habits, taking into account the rhythm preceding the period of incarceration. In this context, *"sexual practices"* refers to any concrete activity closely or remotely related to arousal or its phantasmatic construction. More precisely, it refers to any behavior born of the *search for conscious arousal, obtained from voluntary positive behavior, involving the individual as an actor in the satisfaction of his or her own desire.*

Listening to everyone's narratives, as the *discussions and confessions unfolded,* we saw the emergence of "usual" and "marginal" sexual practices. By choice, and out of a refusal to include any moral judgment in the classification of practices, the terminologies relating to *normality* and *abnormality* seemed prohibitive. The[16] classification here is based solely on a quantitative judgment, bringing to the fore practices which, because they are *commonplace,* have an easier place in collective verbalization. There's a cocktail of modesty and excitement behind the performance of a sexual practice that can only be evoked sparingly, in the presence of selected ears. When prisoners talk about marginal practices, it's taboo. What society does not wish to hear or see, the realities that society forces to be ignored in order to forget them and prevent them from becoming commonplace, which would be detrimental to an established order, but also this culture of silence like a curtain of opprobrium, are the specific characteristics of a sexuality that is kept silent so as not to make it commonplace and accessible. Marginalized practices are inseparable from the silence they imply. This same silence is inseparable from a social system's desire to prevent the proliferation of behaviours that are incompatible with the interests of an established norm to be respected. Taboo rhymes with silence and discretion, rather than prohibition. The freedom that each individual grants himself, to flout the de facto prohibition surrounding the silence of unaccepted practices, demonstrates a particular desire to satisfy a particular need, as well as an ability to distance oneself from a standardized way of functioning in society.

16. These classifications are part of a temporal framework, and presuppose a precise and indestructible interdependence with the contemporary society to which they relate. This is how the typology of sexual needs, sometimes referred to as natural or essential needs, was conceived.

Watertightness, secrets and taboos of a paradoxical institution

To meet the imperative of watertightness, openness to the outside world and to the circumstances of free experience is suppressed, and this is one of the conditions for the continued existence of confinement, as much as one of the constraints of punishment. The institution is built on the principle of a fundamental distance between inside and outside. The use of visiting rooms, forbidden or controlled intimacy, and sexuality seen as a fusion between outside and inside that denies the authority of the institution's walls, are all factors that maintain this power to separate, divide and cleave, like a vestige of the relegation of yesteryear.

In a democracy, giving visibility to prison conditions involves a conflict between two divergent interests. Very often, the transparency of institutions comes up against the imperatives of security. The relative silence and lack of awareness of these malfunctions or dysfunctions is one of the conditions for maintaining the fragile equilibrium that presides over the survival of the institution in its current form. This opacity certainly meets the requirements of a power that cannot show what it cannot be proud of, unless it sets up the violence of vengeance as the punitive mechanism of democratic justice. The veil covering the knowledge of experiences in detention can also be attributed to a society now unaccustomed to the spectacle of torture, whose religious, humanist and republican consciences do not sit well with the endorsement of a prison regime that it is better not to know too much about[17].

Ignorance allows us to avoid individual or collective guilt in the face of this intrinsically imperfect institution, whose replacement is still

---

17. FOUCAULT (Michel), *Surveiller et punir. Naissance de la prison*, Paris, Gallimard, 1975, p. 20.

illusory and unanswerable. Retroactively, the penalty of the past is, still in the present, qualified as barbaric. Today, there's nothing to say that this principle, which has always held true, will escape the qualification of the republican prison of the 20th or 21st century. If it is unthinkable today not to care for and feed prisoners, it will perhaps become incomprehensible for future generations to conceive of the prohibition of sexual relations and the control of pleasures in the broadest sense, in an institution whose punitive vocation is legitimized by the mission of reintegration[18]. Sexuality in prisons is evidence of a meeting point between the reluctance of an institution to reveal what it is, and the reluctance of a population to reveal what it does. Prisons have to hide because they are not always proud of being *too much* and *not enough*. At the same time, when it comes to sexuality, prisoners cannot deny the personal stakes involved in maintaining secrecy.

In prison, everything reminds us that space is enclosed, perpetually fettered by limits. The difficulty of access, the configuration of the premises, the metallic clatter of keys and the clacking of electric locks, punctuate the minutes of every day, and remind us that prison is an insularity conceived by the outside as a perpetual constraint for the inside. Sheltered by its walls and the authority that governs it, the prison is sacralized as a penal tool in the service of justice. However, because its reputation has been tarnished since its inception, and because the legitimacy of the power to punish is being called into question at the same time as the notion of power between individuals is suspected of abuse, domination and submission, respect for the sacred is not self-evident in the prison institution. It must be deduced from the power of an authority that today derives its legitimacy from a dual argument of punishment and rehabilitation.

---

18. FAUGERON (Claude) and LE BOULAIRE (Jean-Michel), *Prisons and prison sentences*, Paris, CESDIP, 1991.

Prison intrinsically assumes that every individual is potentially dishonest and dangerous. Disobedience is its *stock in trade, and it is* from this premise that the many prescriptions of prison life will find their justification. Sexual issues are no exception to this rule; on the contrary, they obey a mechanism of constraint that limits rights with the paradoxical aim of limiting disobedience and illegality. Reducing existences to their lowest common denominator - in this case, the survival of bodies - is also a way of limiting the stakes for an administration whose obligation to achieve results consists primarily in guarding men and women. This is where the prison gets its credibility. Its raison d'être, on the other hand, fluctuates according to penal policy, between dry repression and redemptive punishment. In both cases, those involved in incarceration are well aware that confinement remains "[...] the detestable solution that cannot be avoided"[19].

---

19. Foucault (Michel), *op. cit.* p. 234.

Chapter 2
How to make taboos talk

The present research on sexuality and the prison world is an exercise in the indispensable ability to meet the other in a benevolent neutrality, leaving the *subject-object* ample latitude to be, say and do, without ever eliciting judgment or moralistic appraisal. Sociology requires us to view the other as a *being-existent,* capable of embracing all possibilities in the evocation of his or her experience. Restrictions must be conceived on the basis of a prior definition of the field, and the sociologist must never forget that he or she is voluntarily a listening subject, curious and eager for knowledge and understanding. This essential driving force excludes any submission to disgust, any *a priori* that is not first posited as a hypothesis, but also any censorship on the content of a field that can only be loquacious on condition that it is fully assumed.

Prison micro-society: diversity and uniqueness

With an incarcerated population of 62,420 individuals[20], the prison population represents a diverse cross-section of society, recomposing

---

20. *Statistique mensuelle de la population écrouée et détenue en France au 1ᵉʳ août 2009*, Direction de l'administration pénitentiaire, Bureau des études, de la prospective et des méthodes.

a *micro-society within the* very social entity of which it is a part. The subjects it holds under the power of its walls are the same individuals who outside claim its existence, its raison d'être and its limits. These beings are not representatives of a forbidden outside: they belong to the outside of which they are deprived. Yvan Illitch evokes society's capacity to confine its own people, in one institution or another, with each time, depending on the justifications, thicker or thinner walls, more or less open doors and more or less complex sesames: "Beyond a certain threshold, society becomes a school, a hospital, a prison. Then the great imprisonment begins."[21]

The sample is based mainly on the narratives of men, who represent 95% of the prison population. Women prisoners were also interviewed, and their responses will regularly confirm or refute the analyses. The findings presented here are based primarily on interviews with fifty men in four French detention centers, and eleven women in a single French detention center. In a secondary way, this analysis was confronted with a more informal fieldwork, made up of around seventy men and women, met in a dozen penitentiary establishments located sometimes in Argentina, sometimes in the Philippines and sometimes in Burundi[22].

---

21. ILLITCH (Ivan), in collaboration with GIARD (Luce) and BARDET (Vincent), *La Convivialité*, Paris, Le Seuil, 1973.

22. A survey on the death penalty in Burundi (GAILLARD [Arnaud], "Les couloirs de la mort au Burundi", in *La Peine de mort dans la région des Grands Lacs*, Paris, ECPM, 2008) enabled us to meet some sixty inmates on death row, who were also interviewed in a secondary manner on questions of sexuality. Two trips to Argentina and the Philippines also gave us the opportunity to interview inmates, warders and management staff about their experiences of sexuality in the prisons of Vigan - on Luson Island in the Philippines - and La Plata - in the province of Buenos-Aires. This more informal fieldwork remains an appendix to this analysis, but the observations made outside France, without having the value of a *comparative fieldwork*, have regularly added weight to the analyses of the main fieldwork.

The prison institution is organized around multiple players who, depending on their respective stakes, have their own vision of reality. Thus, this research led to meetings with warders, nurses, a complete psychiatric service, prison directors, rehabilitation staff, inmates' spouses and warders. There were several reasons why it was imperative to extend this field beyond the cell dwellers. Firstly, because prisons are largely unknown, and before relying solely on what inmates have to say, intellectual curiosity was nurtured by a desire to understand and verify. Secondly, because the experience of imprisonment is surrounded by a mythical and historical culture, making it an object that is undoubtedly often rewritten at the whim of those with an interest in it.

In this case, the aim was to bring together a diversity of individuals, in the sense of a *non-discriminatory variety*. In practice, the way in which inmates are recruited differs from one detention center to another. These conclusions relate only to those individuals who were willing, of their own free will, to talk about their sexuality. The discourse of others is absent; so, for lack of reference, it is not possible to qualify, distinguish and analyze the difference between those who agreed to give themselves up, and those who were excluded[23] or refused to be questioned.

In order to objectify the discourse on such an essential theme as sexuality, it was important to meet inmates from all generations, all socio-cultural backgrounds and several different faiths. The identification questions included age, sex, marital status, the existence of offspring, beliefs, rural or urban origin, professional qualifications and occupations held, and finally the reason for conviction, together with

---

23. The management of the Bapaume center has restricted access to certain female prisoners who belonged to the Action directe and ETA movements. These women are subject to the same daily rules of detention, except that all communications with the outside world are subject to special authorization from the prison management.

past and future criminal record, if applicable. The prisoners interviewed had been in prison for between five and twenty-five years[24]. Some of them had previously served several consecutive sentences, interrupted by releases lasting several years.

Some convictions are particularly stigmatizing in terms of social relations within the prison system. However, even if prisons are no longer the world of[25] *kingpins* whose illegalisms remain potential factors of heroism, it was important not to focus this entire study on sex offenders, who are nonetheless increasingly widely represented in French prisons[26]. Inmates were not selected on the basis of their official or unofficial sexual orientation. The interest of this work lies in the deduction of behaviors from a contingent situation, and in the limits of the moral or narcissistic authorization that each person gives himself, to verbalize what is assumed and to keep silent what hurts.

Presumed pitfalls, pitfalls encountered

Starting a field study is not devoid of the exhilarating feeling of adventure that comes with any confrontation with the unknown. We quickly identified three factors that were likely to interfere with the interviews. These were the reticence inherent in the intimate nature of this research, mainly motivated by a *concern for confidentiality*, the *implications of desire* and the *preservation of self-image*. These three types of reluctance can

---

24. Except Stewart and Sly, whom we met in Œrmingen.

25. Here, the words *"caïd"* and *"braqueur" are* regularly used to designate inmates whose offenses and personalities express power and authority, and command admiration in the masculine representations within the *men's prison*. They can be bandits or political prisoners. They are opposed to sex offenders, homosexuals and all kinds of men considered degraded, diminished and submissive.

26. As of July 1st, 2007, the proportion of sex offenders represented 18.8% of convicts in prison. See TOURNIER (Pierre V.), "Arpenter le champ pénal", *Lettre d'information sur les questions pénales*, no. 54, September 10, 2007.

be singular or plural, with effects ranging from *mythomania* to *refusal to answer*. It would be a mistake to describe silence or lies as failures, as these two means of defence in the face of embarrassing questions can, depending on the scale at which they are used, be made talkative once they have been identified. For example, it was to be expected that the guardians of the *men's house*[27], would have some difficulty admitting to unofficial homosexual practices, contrary to an official sexual orientation. Similarly, questions about masturbatory practices and the consequent admission of a feeling of regression, the accessories used in an attempt to reproduce a pleasure or an organ, with self-respect sacrificed to the despair of lack, are all difficult to pronounce. Finally, repeating in front of a stranger the painful confessions made before the judicial authorities, reactivated - especially for sex offenders - a sense of guilt already strongly stimulated on a daily basis, by the stigmatization of pointers within the prison itself.

However, despite these fears, and even if it would be pretentious to claim to have been able to identify all the omissions as well as all the lies[28], the inmates we met played, without surprise, a game they had accepted, knowing the research theme[29]. The gaps now lie in the unknown part of all those anonymous people who were not solicited, or who did not wish to take part in the interviews. While this may enable a precise interpretation of the effects of confinement on sexual

---

27. The expression *maison-des-hommes*, freely borrowed from Maurice Godelier in his study of the Baruyas, is re-used by Daniel Welzer-Lang, Lilian Mathieu and Michaël Faure in *Sexualité et violence en prison*. Here, *maison-des-hommes* refers to prison as a "conservatory of masculine values", rather than an institution promoting a process of learning masculinity like military service.

28. At the end of the interview, each person was asked to specify whether the need to lie had arisen: the attitude of the answer was undoubtedly more eloquent than its verbalized content.

29. With the exception of two Travellers we met in Saint-Mihiel, where the deputy director chose not to announce that it was a research project on sexuality.

personalities, it is the limitation of a study based mainly on qualitative analysis, which cannot claim to be exhaustive in terms of representation of a population.

Anyone coming from outside is welcomed into the prison as a *breath of fresh air*, a sign that life beyond the walls is still alive. This premise gave the encounters during these interviews a positive *a priori*. When it's not a question of a reciprocal and reversible relationship of desire between interviewee and interviewer, the pitfall of sociological interviews is sometimes a relationship of identification. Both desire and identification give rise to a concern to please in order not to displease. To please the other in the otherness of desire, and to please oneself in that the interviewer represents a mirror echoing a reality of oneself, brought to life by the sudden projection of words. The difficulty lies in the nature of the feeling that animates both the speaker and the listener. Anne-Marie Marchetti expresses this sentiment when she introduces her work on long sentences[30]. Psychoanalytic terminology, when it deals with the transfer of feelings that may arise between the analysand and the analysed under the notion of *transference*, is not far removed from the practice of sociological interviews, all the more so when the latter deal with intimacy and sexuality. We had to be particularly vigilant about the interactions that can arise through desire and sentimental expressions of affection or hostility, seduction or rejection, during these individual interviews conducted in the discretion of a visiting room. Depending on the gender of the individuals interviewed, their age and culture, as well as the reason for their conviction and the stigma attached to sexual offending, the interviews generate representations for both the interviewer and the interviewee that are no strangers to *who they are*. In maintaining the delicate balance between "commitment"

---

30. MARCHETTI (Anne-Marie), *op. cit.* p. 12.

and "distancing" referred to by Norbert Elias, the researcher is also a player in these multiple encounters[31].

The issue of confidentiality arose in connection with narratives that could be construed as an admission of disciplinary misconduct. It should be remembered that, in judicial matters, verbalisation is synonymous with confession. The imperatives necessitated by the fear of the authority's power to punish, hierarchically supplant the mechanisms for protecting privacy. This observation endorses the power of prison authority and its power to punish. When the treasures of intimacy are easier to reveal than any narrative suggesting possible punishment, it's because discipline, like a sword of Damocles, possesses a power to impress that we would be wrong to confuse with the power to dissuade. It's not a question of *not doing*, it's a question of *not saying*, because words that are often said to liberate, are sometimes also false friends who lock you up. Detention is a hostile and violent environment, in which it is always preferable to develop avoidance behaviors in the face of situations, rather than having to develop genuine means of defense when conflict arises. When, in the end, the desire to tell the truth overcame the fear of confession, two conclusions emerged. On the one hand, the sociologist's function inspires a confidence that sets him apart from the prison administration. On the other hand, speaking out, when risky, remains an act of resistance.

The priority choice of speech

As soon as the content of the discourse, or the circumstances in which it takes place, can be shown to play a part in the stakes of the *place one wishes to occupy*, or *the place in which one refuses to be placed,*

---

31. ELIAS (Norbert), *Engagement et distanciation. Contributions à la sociologie de la connaissance*, Paris, Fayard, 1993, p. 9.

then words are no longer reliable. Answers are perceived as self-assessments, based on criteria whose assumed and accepted power consists in ranking one's own singularity within the social group. Sociological research presupposes, as a preamble to any analysis, a certainty of having been understood by the subjects in the field. The prison population includes illiterate individuals, and others whose cultural level undoubtedly does not allow them to grasp the intelligibility expected from the questioning. We quickly opted for semi-structured interviews, transcribed by manual note-taking. Far beyond passive or participant observation, and from the point of view of the interviewee, the interviews turned out to be confessions that were always generous, and sometimes relieving. This interplay of interests reminds us that, in all circumstances, the sociologist is a subject among subjects, and that without this recognition, sociology runs the risk of theorizing below or above what it wishes to make clear, while at the same time engaging in this quest for meaning turned towards what Jan Spurk defines as a "more optimistic future"[32].

Beyond the verbal, the practice of interviewing allows us to recover a wealth of information which, in subtext, confirms or refutes the grammatical content of the discourse. Because experience hides beyond words, in attitudes, intonations, smiles, tremors, tears and laughter, it would have been illusory to be satisfied with a quantitative survey based on questionnaires. However, the questionnaire method was used to interview warders and inmates' spouses.

In *face-to-face communication,* any behavior is likely to represent a response, from the moment the slightest silence, the slightest rictus or eyelid twitch can be interpreted, at least unconsciously, by the person

---

32. Spurk (Jan), *Quel avenir pour la sociologie*, Paris, PUF, 2006, p. 188.

dialoguing. Even if the development of defense mechanisms can act as a brake on sincerity, language is not limited to words organized according to the grammar of a language. Beyond the ideas uttered and like the action of a *stimulus*, listening rarely leaves you impassive. Taboos are certainly easier to verbalize when they appear behind the complete anonymity of a written questionnaire. Yet the cause of this disadvantage is also an advantage. The listener's ear is also aided by the eyes and all that makes up the *self* in the role of being the *other* for the interlocutor. The fear of being judged feeds on the same things as the fear of being found out when you lie, embellish or omit. The face-to-face interview is therefore particularly interesting for the relationship it establishes.

When it comes to sexuality, quantitative surveys can be hazardous. The cultural stakes for each gender are diametrically opposed. Where men overestimate the value of their masculine attributes, according to cultural criteria that require them to embody power, women underestimate the value of their femininity, culturally sanctioned by the image of potential motherhood that imposes restraint. Whatever the tools chosen to explore issues of sexuality sociologically, any study of this kind elicits schizophrenic reactions. Challenges to the credibility of the field approach are matched by undiminished interest when it comes to delving into the results of the survey. It's as if sexuality, although viewed through the prism of sociology, possessed a power that was as attractive as it was repulsive, reminiscent of the tandem of desire and prohibition that is widespread in the mindset[33].

---

33. Bozon (Michel), "Observer l'inobservable : la description et l'analyse de l'activité sexuelle", *in* Bajos (Nathalie) *et al,* (sous la direction de), *Sexualité et sida,* Paris, Agence nationale de recherches sur le sida, December 1995, p. 43.

Sites analyzed

Assuming that the *duration* parameter is an inescapable element in the study of the experience of incarceration, this research therefore implied taking an interest only in long sentences[34], thus excluding remand prisons[35] where overcrowding conditions are often criticized. Similarly, central prisons, whose purpose is to house *dangerous* or *difficult* inmates, and whose access is considered particularly risky due to reinforced security measures, were excluded. This study therefore focuses on the particularities of five detention centers, governed by the *numerus clausus* principle and individual cell confinement. Interviewees were recruited in consultation with the management of the centers concerned, sometimes on the basis of a posting in detention, sometimes on the basis of an invitation by post without specifying the research topic, sometimes on the basis of a selection made by the prison administration, and sometimes on the personal initiative of inmates.

In practice, the extent to which people are allowed to experience sexuality varies not only from facility to facility, but also according to the gender of the detainee population. Each facility therefore has its own specific characteristics. What's more, inmates are often the actors in these divergent regimes. When it comes to long sentences, it's important to remember that although the prison governor is the prison authority, he or she is transferred more frequently than the individuals in his or her charge. The atmosphere and prerogatives acquired by the *law of numbers* therefore sometimes fall more on the

---

34. In penal establishments, and particularly in detention centers, a *long sentence* means more than five years. This is the minimum length of time observed in the field study.
35. In principle, prisons are reserved for pre-trial detainees or for sentences and residual sentences of less than one year.

prison population than on the administration that governs it. So, as they move from one center to another, inmates are aware of the reputations that circulate and differentiate establishments despite common legal references.

SECOND PART

LIVING YOUR SEXUALITY IN PRISON
- *The missing otherness* -

> "Sexual activity is thus part of the broad horizon of death and life, of time, becoming and eternity. It is made necessary because the individual is doomed to die, and so that in some way he escapes death."[36]

Marital relationships, and therefore emotional and family relationships in general, and sexuality in particular, are an axial denominator of all existence. What about those whose mirrors reflect only gray walls, inhabited by individuals of the same sex, with whom all conjugal sexuality is prohibited? What about those who leave behind in the visiting room a person they dream of cherishing every day, and for whom the anguish of "deception" and separation haunts every return from the visiting room, every letter received, every phone call? The gaps left by the impossible carnal encounter with this *chosen other* are a disturbance in the prison experience. This is in addition to the loss of freedom, the confinement, the monosexual universe and the impossibility of organizing an existence according to a chosen perspective.

In sexual terms, prison represents a deprivation of otherness whose influence is not unrelated to the length of the sentence. Starting from

36. FOUCAULT (Michel), *Histoire de la sexualité II. L'usage des plaisirs*, Paris, Gallimard, coll. "Tel", 1984, p. 178.

an identification of the singularity of sexual needs, the aim is to analyze the adaptations developed in the circumstances of this absence of the other, which leads to solitary sexual practices. What is the nature of the lack felt? Is it mainly a lack of self-recognition, due to the impossibility of seducing the opposite sex? Or is it the carnal involvement of the physical organs that reminds us of the certainty of our own existence, in our relationship with the other and in the experience of pleasure? Where does sexuality begin? With a mixing of bodies, or with an encounter between beings who combine a desire, more or less equivalent, to consume acts of sexual excitement together?

Chapter 1
The singularity of sexual needs

To understand the influence of sexuality during imprisonment in a monosexual world, we need to assess the importance of sexuality for each of the individuals we interviewed, from the perspective of a comparative look at life before and during imprisonment. Among the many accounts of life in detention, sexuality is either omnipresent or summarily absent. There's a divide between those inmates who feel the need to address the issue of difficult or even impossible sexual relationships because they are forbidden, and those whose silence is all the more questioning because it frustrates a question that everyone is asking. There are a number of possible explanations for this phenomenon identified during the interviews. It's true that when it comes to talking about intimacy, modesty and reserve are obstacles. However, since the interviews were conducted on the basis of a prior adherence to the sociological object presented[37], the eagerness to talk about lacks, the hatred expressed in the face of this denial of sexual needs, and the words used to describe adaptation to the prohibition of sexual relations, prompt us to apprehend the different intensities of discourse, based

---

37. With the exception of the Saint-Mihiel detention center near Verdun, where the deputy director wrote to inmates inviting them to take part in interviews on prison life, without specifying the subject of the research.

on the notion of "sexual needs", for which three ideal-types have been identified.

Assessing sexual needs: a de facto inequality

Without going into psychological or physiological explanations, which would attempt to rationalize the quantity of a libidinal need, it seemed important to evaluate, for each of the interviewees, the importance of sexuality alternately with regard to experiences outside and inside. Thus, independently of the experience of sexuality in detention, the interviews focused on verbalizing the discovery of sexuality in adolescence, solitary and couple practices, the place that sexuality might have taken in life prior to incarceration and, finally, adaptation to the restrictive conditions of sexuality in detention.

Contrary to Sigmund Freud's conclusion that "sexual life does not begin at puberty, but manifests itself much earlier after birth"[38], the inmates were first asked about the age at which masturbation began, the circumstances of this discovery, the circumstances of the practices during their lives (alone or with others), and finally the frequency, observing three different periods: adolescence, adulthood at liberty, and the time of incarceration.

As masturbation is understood here as a type of sexual practice in its own right, the use of this practice has been alternatively analyzed either as the continuation of a specific practice existing outside, or as the coping mechanism of a lack of sexual relationship to be compensated for. In this sense, the study of masturbation frequency alone cannot be understood as a factor determining the quantity of the need for

---

38. FREUD (Sigmund), *op. cit.* p. 13.

sexuality. The frequency studied was also put into perspective with the frequency of sexual relations between couples prior to incarceration. The analysis also focused on the variety of sexual experiences, the number of partners, the freedom and enthusiasm to evoke sexual memories, and the fact of identifying, in a couple relationship, the most demanding person. The qualitative and quantitative importance of sexuality is therefore determined on the basis of a range of weighted elements.

A typology of sexual needs

Beyond reproductive objectives, sexual needs represent a search for pleasure, a confrontation with otherness and the expression of feelings whose necessity fluctuates according to each individual. This management of sexual needs distinguishes the human species from other animal species, according to individual elaborations which are not without influence on the singularities of the experience of sexuality in detention[39]. Thus, for each individual, sexuality takes on necessities that are not unrelated to the intensity of need, which directly governs the intensity of lack. Three different types of sexual need have thus been identified, determining three ways of considering sexuality in individual existence, but also three ways of enduring the contingency of monosexual confinement and the prohibition of sexual relations within detention: the *non-substitutable vital need*, the *substitutable circumstantial need*, and the *cancellable moderate need*. For each of these needs, the quantity of sexuality, the sexuality/feeling tandem and the benefits derived from sexual practice are different. The consequences of incarceration will, in fact, vary according to the person's experience of the sexual rupture caused by incarceration.

---

39. On the distinction between human desires and instincts, see KANT (Emmanuel), *Anthropologie du point de vue pragmatique*, Paris, Flammarion, 1993, tome III, p. 217.

The vital, non-substitutable need: "No more fucking means nothing!"

Sexuality is experienced as a need, in the form of a non-pathological addiction. From their earliest sexual practices, these individuals have demanded that their bodies satisfy a desire several times a day. This masturbatory frequency in adolescence continues with a similar frequency of sexual relations. Unless they find a partner capable of satisfying needs of identical intensity, these individuals will satisfy themselves with multiple partners, in a way that is as free as it is guilt-free. Sexuality is not necessarily an obsession in the pathological sense of the term, but a quantitatively important need, the intensity of which requires frequent practice.

Sexuality is described as a leisure activity, a passion practiced intensely, for the benefit of well-being and a feeling of completeness. Satisfaction is not viewed here solely in terms of quantity. Sexuality is just as much appreciated as it is delightful. The qualitative dimension is therefore sought by these lovers of *good sex* who recognize themselves as renowned lovers. The search for new partners also seems to be facilitated by a reputation that precedes them. There is not necessarily conjugality, but a conjugation of interests focused exclusively on satisfying a desire for pleasure. The idea of possession is not preponderant in these lovers; respect for the other necessarily implies a dimension of freedom, in this case that of playing the same game with a variety of partners seeking the same enjoyment. The discourse of these individuals seems to corroborate the hypothesis of an intimate and inevitable conjugation between body and mind, between physiological and psychological equilibrium, between bodily satisfaction and the expectations of a self that cannot be forgotten, as Paul Schilder concludes: "The individual would be working towards his own death if the libidinal tendencies did not take care to preserve the integrity of the organism: they divert the destructive tendency of the subject onto the object [...]".[40]

One of the parameters for identifying this vital, non-substitutable need is the ease with which alternative sexual practices can be evoked as an assumed normality. Guilt and society's view of the marginality of these practices have no hold. The freedom enjoyed by these individuals is also expressed in the search for new experiences. Freedom does not mean the desire to try everything, but the open possibility of tasting hitherto unknown pleasures, likely to extend the possibilities of satisfaction in search of novelty as much as perfection. It's a need that knows little or no self-censorship. This ideal type implies a very precise conception of expectations and needs. This can be seen in the prison environment, with *visiting companions*[41], friends of friends, who come to visit particular inmates, implicitly assuming the sexual satisfaction they will offer and obtain. The conjugal relationship is essentially based on an exchange of pleasure between consenting individuals. Nothing is negotiated, nothing is exchanged for money; it's an unspoken contract born of the mutual acceptance of a personal pleasure acquired with the participation of the other's pleasure.

The experience of sexuality during incarceration therefore appears to be a major problem for these interviewees, whose sexuality is as *demanding* in quality as it is in quantity. In prison, these individuals feel that their impulses and their very being are curbed. As sexual practice is one of their major and often daily desires, sexual deprivation is akin to the deprivation of an element essential to their existence as much as to their sustenance. The regime imposed by incarceration is experienced as a punishment added on to the deprivation of liberty. It is all the more

---

40. SCHILDER (Paul), *L'Image du corps*, Paris, Gallimard, 1980.
41. Expression used by the inmates themselves.

difficult for these inmates to maintain the continuity of their being within the prison walls, the greater the rupture. A weaning mechanism is required, in order to persist in being inside what they were outside. What happens to an inveterate swimmer when the water suddenly becomes forbidden? The necessary compensation for a practice with multiple objectives: "To fuck is to be. To fuck no more is to be nothing." Ryan explains how this daily need is throbbing, and awakens at the slightest solicitation: "Once you've had sex, you need it again and again, it's like a drug. Here I jerk off every day. It's a huge craving, especially when the matrons come, I want to touch their breasts."

Prisoners' anger at the experience of incarceration is intimately linked to sexual deprivation. This feeling is all the stronger where sexual needs are concerned. There's a sense of *dispossession of an essential,* which makes the regime of sexuality in detention a particularly punitive provision. Because they experience little self-censorship, individuals whose sexual needs are vital and unsubstitutable used to diversify their sexual practices outside prison. On the contrary, the constraint of imprisonment restricts the range of possible practices. Léon, incarcerated in Val-de-Reuil, declares: "I've always enjoyed being an exhibitionist. [...] I'm open to all sexual practices, because there's always someone you can meet who's ready for the same delirium."

Others combined sexual and financial satisfaction in a professionalization of their sexuality. This is the case of Marcus, detained in Val-de-Reuil: "I was a sex professional, making private films and *peep shows.* I even practiced zoophilia for a film where I masturbated a dog. I hated it..."

Here, sexuality is perceived as inseparable from existence. Expressed in the form of a prerogative, it is an elementary right supposedly inalienable, whose capture by the prison institution leaves a feeling of injustice, all the more indigestible as it rests on the paradox of an unspoken fact. These individuals develop legal, historical and social arguments, combining knowledge of the prohibition with demands. Since sexuality is a particularly important issue for them, their thoughts on incarceration cannot ignore a problem that is of secondary importance to others. This is the case for Tony, who sees the deprivation of sexual relations as a way of establishing domination over the inmate population, albeit at a price to be paid in terms of human resources management: "If we could get laid, the prison administration would have fewer problems. But in fact they prefer to frustrate us to show us that we're no longer the boss, that we're guided and restrained completely."

Deprivation is such a source of frustration that abstinence is unthinkable. These prisoners organize meetings in the visiting room, where they *consume sex*[42]. Nothing can replace the satisfaction of this libido. Masturbation and the use of pornography are not sufficient palliatives. However, the frequency of masturbation can be as high as ten times a day, depending on the discourse and circumstances. During a stay in solitary confinement, these inmates find themselves alone, with no other social referent than themselves or the warden who serves them their meals, and confess to masturbating to the point of injuring their genitals, even though they are already used to the intense pace. Personal equilibrium is at stake, and every effort will be made to circumvent the de facto difficulties imposed by the prison regime.

These inmates have a point of view on pointers mixed with indulgence and disgust. Their open-minded approach to sexual practices enables them to deal with the problems highlighted by sexual offences in a calm

---

42. Insofar as laxity is allowed by the detention center that takes them in. However, it should be noted that those individuals whose sexual needs are vital and unsubstitutable are the most daring to defy the prohibitions.

manner. Nevertheless, they themselves have sometimes suffered sexual violence as children, and the mere idea that their own libertinism might equate them with pointers is unbearable for them. They are quick to describe pointers as sick, perverted and unhinged, to be distrusted by society. Their severity is more focused on the punishment they wish to see inflicted on them, than on the consideration given to them in their day-to-day dealings. This attitude is pragmatic, as the desire to remove a recognized danger to society is not sustained by a feeling of disgust that feeds a poisonous climate in detention.

The circumstantial substitutable need: "I make do with what I have on hand!"

This sexual need is that of prisoners whose libido is closely dependent on the circumstances of their existence. It oscillates between a *necessary* and an *accessory aspect*: because sexuality is generally less important, there are circumstances where it doesn't matter. This does not prevent these individuals from being very demanding in circumstances where sexuality is possible. In terms of prison-related grievances, the lack of relationships is not mentioned as a priority. In fact, the sexual theme is evoked by words belonging more to the register of tenderness and sentimental relationships. Sexuality corresponds to the attribute of an affective relationship, and the search for otherness is satisfied above all by sharing the other as both a *loving* and *desiring being*.

The sexual relations evoked are the object of an encounter in which the "unmastered" is the subject of doubt and fear. Sexual practice is deduced from the adult's place in the social world. It is part of the attributes of being, but not consciously an axial element. On the other hand, the partner's plasticity is of particular importance. In the seduction mechanism, there's a search for self-love, interdependent with a narcissistic posture expressed in hushed tones. The relationship with the other is nourished by a preoccupation with appearance, with the quest to belong to a social model in which these inmates seek a reflection of who they are as they want to be. Many showed particular concern for maintaining their ability to seduce, through a preoccupation with coquetry ranging from clothing to sculpting their bodies *through* body-building, hairstyling or make-up for women. Purely sexual frustration is soothed by palliatives such as masturbation, often associated with pornography, which replaces the erotic imagery lacking in a monosexual world. Masturbation is practiced under conditions and with frequencies reminiscent of the adolescent period. So it's only natural that sexual relations should be replaced by solitary practices, reminiscent of periods when couple relationships were rare or non-existent.

The lack of sexual relations is at the level of affect, whose interdependence with sexuality, while not obligatory, is here almost systematic. Tom, an inmate at Œrmingen, explains: "Sexuality begins when there's love, and we start kissing." Moreover, a mix occurs in the discourse on objects of affect. The questioning of sexuality transits towards the search for tenderness with a partner, to finally reach the evocation of the lack of filial affective sharing. Prison is thus an obstacle to maintaining family relationships, before being an obstacle to sexual pleasure. The resulting frustration is experienced in a different way: the impossibility of being a *lover* or *parent* comes before the impossibility of being a *lover*. Sexual deprivation in prison does not, therefore, include the dimension of physical lack as a priority argument. Tom, who claims to have had four partners in his entire life, puts it into perspective: "You can live without it just fine. I make do with what I have on hand. Some people do nothing, like priests and divorcees for that matter. Others let off steam with violence."

Of course, incarceration castrates the ability to seduce, to love and be loved, but the hardship of sexual deprivation is not necessarily due to the contingencies of confinement. Tom continues: "I haven't been able to have sex since my divorce, because I still loved my ex-wife. With her, we did it three times a week, or even every day when we weren't tired. I can't live for myself. So since my wife left me, I've been living for my son, and that's enough to keep me from going crazy."

These inmates don't necessarily have an elaborate discourse on the prohibition of sexuality, and are sometimes even genuinely surprised to hear the word *"prohibition" mentioned*. They are indulgent in their acceptance of this reality. Sexual deprivation has historically been part of punishment. No matter where it comes from, no matter what is allowed in other countries, only one thing is certain: sexuality and prison don't *mix*. The deprivation of sexuality is induced, assumed and therefore tacitly accepted, as a social rather than a legal rule: "Of course you don't fuck in prison!" Wolf, whom we met outside after his release, and for whom "prison is nothing other than the mirror of the society in which it is embedded", describes the circumstantial aspect of his sexual need as follows: "I'm not going to change my life in depth, my way of breathing or my way of living because I'm in prison. I'm restricted in what I can do, but you have to do what you can outside, that is, with the possibilities you have. I'm not going to torture my mind by talking or thinking all the time about something I can't do."

When it comes to answering questions about sexual development in detention, the answer invariably involves describing a place for emotional and/or family reunion. The sexual dimension is often avoided, or expressed only in passing. The intimate nature of sexuality is seen as a means of protecting it, as the guarantee of a possession that is kept secret so as not to lose it. To allow the prison institution to interfere with sexual satisfaction is to place sexuality in the public arena, to lose protective intimacy and to feel an obligation to perform, fuelled by potential competition. So there's a kind of tacit acceptance of the current situation imposed by the prison regime. These inmates spoke of sexual breakdowns, the impossibility of practicing sexuality in this or that circumstance, the need to be reassured by a controlled framework in order to access sexual pleasure serenely. Paradoxically, these same inmates speak of lack in a tone close to the conditional and hypothetical. The consequences of deprivation are assumed rather than deduced. The question of resuming sexuality on leaving prison is never expressed. It is probably understood more as the resumption of an affective relationship from which the sexual relationship will be deduced. This gives rise to the myth of the prison leaver, notably embodied by Jeanne Moreau in *Les Valseuses*[43], whose first and ultimate necessity is to "get laid". Wolf recounts: "I resumed sexual relations with my girlfriend two weeks after my release.

Despite the rupture effect, in a dynamic of survival and maintenance of *self-existence*, the libido in this ideal-type takes on a more or less controlled and conscious face, the consequences of which are not to be overlooked. Hatred of the institution, of life, of society, the psychic imbalances that can result from the deprivation of sexual relations are not excluded. Quite simply, these inmates pretend to divert at least part of their sexual needs. This does not prevent Jacques Lesage de La Haye[44] from analyzing the consequences of lack and frustration as follows: "Sexual frustration makes you violent. [...] And it's also to say that the work of lamination of the prison in relation to emotional and sexual frustration is such that it ends up making people unconsciously mad, desperate, consumed by hatred and driven by desires for revenge.

---

43. *Les Valseuses*, film by Bertrand Blier, France, 1974.
44. Jacques Lesage de La Haye is a former prisoner. During his eleven years of incarceration, he studied psychology, became a doctor of psychology, then obtained a chair at the University of Paris Saint-Denis. He is a member of the GIP (Groupe d'information sur les prisons) with Michel Foucault, and continues to host a weekly program, *Ras les murs*, on Radio Libertaire.

Living your sexuality in prison - the missing otherness -

[...] On the surface, they become good prisoners-citizens-adapted, but inside, they're in a very bad way."

Here, the criticism of the pointers is mostly justified by the concern to protect conjugal entities and children. Something akin to respect for the family unit, seen as a social entity whose model is reassuring. Hence a particular severity in judging these fellow inmates, with whom a form of ostracism is practiced that seems to act as a transference of hatred: "It's all the difference between metabolizing one's own hatred to make it a subversive factor, a factor of adaptation, or repressing it within oneself by pretending that one has overcome it like a magnificent hero, and in fact finding a very subtle way of communicating it to others so that others are acted upon by this unspoken hatred."[45]

Cancellable moderate need: "I've never been into the thing."

Sexuality is presented here as a secondary preoccupation, both inside and out. Sometimes arriving late in life, sexual practices are also rare in terms of quantity. Masturbation appears to be a compulsory part of adolescence, arrived at through *generational identification*. However, after the "what's done is done" effect, these individuals have gone through the phases specific to each individual's development, with very moderate enthusiasm. It's not necessarily a question of an absence of sexuality, even if that's the category into which *virgins* would be classified, but of an avowed detachment from all forms of sexuality, which is never evoked as an inherent need of existence. The sexual desert is sometimes accompanied by a sentimental desert, in which phases of solitude and celibacy alternate with affective relationships in equal proportions. The number of sentimental relationships is reduced, and unless forced, the frequency of sexual practices during a couple's relationship is monthly rather than weekly. The number of partners in a lifetime is reported

---

45. GAILLARD (Arnaud), *Interview with Jacques Lesage de La Haye*, Paris, 2005.

to be less than ten, or even less than five, without any moral censure. Geronimo confides: "I've only had three female partners in my life, and I've only had about twenty sexual relationships in all. I don't miss it, because I was sickened by sex when I was raped as a kid."

Sex is mainly perceived as an accessory to the sentimental relationship, whose constitution is essentially based on relationships of tenderness potentially devoid of eroticism. Sex is also limited to the reproductive dimension. Because sexual desires frequently disappear due to the contingency of incarceration, there is no need to substitute a new form of sexual practice for the prohibition or impossibility of conjugal relations. The sexual need is cancelled out in prison, just as it could have been, or had already been, cancelled out outside. The rupture effect of incarceration appears less significant than for the previous two ideal-types. It stems from the inmates' discourse, which reveals a sexual desire and practices that are more or less identical between *pre-incarceration*, the sexuality of the outside world, and *during incarceration*, the sexuality of the inside world. As Françoise, an inmate at Bapaume, puts it: "I've never been into the whole thing, so I don't miss it at all. I'm even better off here in prison, because outside, it's my husband who always wanted to."

Prisoners, whose needs are moderate and annulable, present particular difficulties in understanding sexual offences; they are "sick". Pathologization is the only acceptable rational approach. As a result, their feelings towards the pointers emanate more from pity than hatred. The situation is beyond them, and mixing *conventional offenders* with *sex offenders* in the same detention center is felt to be an aberration and a humiliation.

When the mind recalls that the body has needs, however rare, masturbation will be experienced as a sufficient solution, also in reduced quantities: less than once a month, if ever. Nono, an inmate at Saint-Mihiel, explains: "I masturbate naturally, but quite rarely. I've never been one for it. It happened to me outside that I didn't meet a woman for over three years. That was after a separation, and the descent into hell that followed. [...] I masturbate once a month in front of Ciné Frisson, to check that the machine is working, but without seeking pleasure."

What's more, since they have little desire or conscious fantasy to achieve arousal, they use pornography as a quasi-material aid for mechanical masturbation. So it's not so much an absence of sexuality as a dormant sexuality, the cause of which is not solely attributed to the contingency of the monosexual universe. The wishes for change in the current visiting room system also focus on reconstituting family ties, without ever raising the question of carnal intimacy. In fact, sexuality is inconceivable within prison walls. It's not so much an uncondi-tional submission to the institution as a tacit acceptance of temporary deprivation as the expression of an offence for which they frequently acknowledge responsibility. At the same time, these inmates declare themselves dominated both in life and in their sexual relationships. This is the case of Geronimo, who, at 34, has already spent fourteen years in prison, with several convictions. He was raped in prison, and finds himself deprived of a woman he married while in custody, and with whom he has never been able to practice coitus. His opinion of prison was particularly indulgent, given the price he seems to have already paid to the institution: "In the end, prison teaches you to be human, it's positive in the long term, it takes away the desire to re-offend. But in the short term, you get out and do anything. You rebuild yourself in prison, if you stay long enough, and you deconstruct yourself if you don't stay long enough."

Chapter 2
The stakes of desire
in monosexual confinement

Upon hearing the subject of this research, inmates regularly exclaimed, "But there's no sexuality in prison!" This response appears to be an exculpatory defense to the evocation of compensatory practices that are sometimes difficult to assume. Removing sex from language is a way of controlling it, mastering it, managing its deprivation and silencing its substitutes.

The deprivation of sexual relations

> "The deprivation of sexual relations [...] is the worst form of corporal punishment, it's torture. What I find crazy is that then, after fifteen years, they'll make you go in front of a shrink to see if you're not too damaged and if they can let you out."[46]

The ban on sexual relations and the denial of conjugal relationships lead male and female prisoners to reconstruct their sexuality on the basis of a virtualized otherness, or materialized by objects whose use can

---

46. MARCHETTI (Anne-Marie), *op. cit.* p. 230.

only be justified in a situation of lack. Reconstituting the other when you're alone is the challenge imposed by the prison administration. Sexuality in detention thus takes on many faces, and opens the way to multiple analyses. Michel Foucault evoked the perpetuation of corporal punishment that had simply taken on a different face. In keeping with the terrain encountered, this is the angle from which the deprivation of sexual relations is viewed here: "The body, according to this penality, is caught up in a system of constraint and deprivation, obligation and prohibition. [Punishment has gone from an art of unbearable sensations to an economy of suspended rights"[47]

Experiencing deprivation

"Being sexually frustrated for years does not improve the individual. It only aggravates his weaknesses."[48]

Questions of discipline, violence, suicide, domination, physical and psychological health, are all indicators of an interest in the sexuality of bodies that die when they no longer exult. Sexuality is mainly seen as the evocation of coital relations, of practices leading to orgasm. The whole psychological and social dimension is abstracted from an approach revolving around the genital, the forbidden, the taboo and the intimate. Before talking about sexual issues, the inmate population expresses a whole series of lacks and sufferings, assuming that their discourse has no connection with the object of this study. It's as if talking about sexuality had to contain the word *"sex" in* order to be precisely targeted. Thus, the issues of affectivity, tenderness and feelings of loneliness are cited before any sexual claims. The majority of the detainee population

---

47. FOUCAULT (Michel), *Surveiller et punir. Naissance de la prison*, Paris, Gallimard, 1975, p. 16.
48. LESAGE DE LA HAYE (Jacques), *La Guillotine du sexe. La vie affective et sexuelle des prisonniers*, Paris, L'Atelier/Éditions Ouvrières, 1998, p. 219.

declare that they do not identify any sexual disturbance. For the men, to do otherwise would be to confess to physiological problems suggesting an impotence that is impossible to verbalize, except in Bruno's pessimistic words: "You can survive anything thanks to masturbation, but it's disturbing and it's going to generate new behavior, blockages, impotence, or an appetite for other things, which will lead you back to prison... In the end, it's like a dog on a leash."

And yet, during imprisonment, the amount of libido seems to fluctuate, recalling periods of deficiency previously experienced on the outside. This discourse is equally shared by men and women, even if the stakes of admitting to a damaged sexuality seem particularly different for male and female *egos* respectively: the loss of desire in men is experienced as a disappearance of virile power. Depending on the sexual needs defined above, the tension accumulated over years of deprivation remains a problem that some manage to cope with through masturbation and pornographic consumption, while others evoke a growing lack of tenderness and affection, summing up their existence in a throbbing rhythm of work, meals and sleep.

For women who, for the most part, declare that they never masturbate, the accumulation of unsatisfied desires has no other outlet than an intensification of expressions of tenderness and affection in front of a man with whom they project themselves in an unconditional and fantasized way. Nanou, a prisoner in Bapaume, beaten by all the men in her life, describes her relationship with her new husband, whom she met while in prison: "When it comes to sex, I've always been a bit forced. As a couple, I was frigid and cold, and as I took a beating every time, there was no foreplay. [...] My new husband's photos are everywhere. I have urges, I'm craving penetration. I need to make love. [...] With him, that's no longer a problem, I'm guaranteed happiness."

Sexual deprivation is not a lack of orgasms, but rather a degradation of self-image due to a lack of interaction between the self and otherness. It is also the affective dimension frequently associated with sexual relations that is lacking, plunging inmates into a feeling of existential solitude. The lack of sexual relations places everyone in a relationship of supply and demand in a market in which the body is a commodity. The impact of lack of sexual relations is relativized in terms of freedom, while it remains significant in terms of otherness. Geronimo, whom we met in Val-de-Reuil, speaks of his ability to be free in *spite of everything*: "We always manage to create a minimum of freedom for ourselves, spiritual freedom, mental freedom...".

Even if in prison, as in other forms of totalitarianism, as Hannah Arendt explained[49], there are still forms of resistance that attest to the fact that psychic life is never completely destroyed, tenderness and sexuality cannot truly exist without the presence of that other who is missing. And if the deprivation of freedom is accepted as an intrinsic part of the very foundation of incarceration, the deprivation of sexual relations is widely seen as an accessory consequence, albeit one with main effects, bordering on illegality, as Alain Monnereau puts it: "The non-sexuality of incarcerated people is just one of the many aspects of the lawlessness in which every prisoner is locked up".[50]

The principle of non-compensation

"The state of barbarism differs from civilization in two characteristic features: 1o in the strength of irascible appetites; 2o in the small

---

49. Arendt (Hannah), *The Origins of Totalitarianism*, Paris, Le Seuil, 1998
50. Monnereau (Alain), *La Castration pénitentiaire*, Paris, Lumière et Justice, 1986, p. 14.

number of objects of enjoyment which offer themselves to concupiscible appetites."[51]

To the question: "How do you compensate for the deprivation of sexual relations?" the answer invariably is that, since a relationship presupposes at least two partners, there is no possible compensation in prison. For women, the discourse on sexuality is largely free of a certain number of issues, such as the expression of power and self-esteem. That's why the equation imposed by lack is more commonly accepted: "Not being desired ends up persuading you to stop being desirable", as women put it. "Not being able to penetrate will persuade you to become impotent", as men will say. In the end, because compensation is prevented, it's the granting of leave that appears in the majority of cases as a response to the ban on sexual relations, or more broadly, as a way of renewing affective ties. Younger inmates seemed more inclined to seize the opportunity of furloughs to seduce and consume sex, while older inmates were more into a staged seduction process that would not lead to sexual practices as part of a temporary release. Others spoke of visits to prostitutes as a recreational and reassuring sexual practice, allowing them to wait months longer for their next parole. This is the case of Ford, detained in Œrmingen: "At the moment, I have a leave every fortnight. I go to Germany to see prostitutes... But you mustn't repeat this... Normally, I'm not allowed to leave the country. But in the end, I'm disturbed by this obligation to pay a woman I'm sleeping with. Yet I've already tried to have a normal relationship on perm, but it's too short to seduce."

These practices are *therapeutic in terms of* restoring the certainty of proper functioning of the genital organs. They are *liberating* when it

---

51. BENTHAM (Jeremy), *Traité de législation civile et pénale*, Paris, Rey et Gravier, 1830, tome II, p. 42.

comes to rediscovering pleasure for two, which definitely doesn't bring the same sensations as solitary pleasure. They are *frustrating* when it comes to the need to alleviate existential loneliness, through the complicity of two beings based on the satisfaction of a common and similar interest.

Prisoners talk about creating a schedule that leaves no time for thought, and that exhausts the body. It's a quest for stupefaction that some also find through psychotropic drugs, and that others organize by accumulating professional, sporting and associative activities: "I can't compensate, I miss it, so I keep busy so that I'm tired in the evening."[52] Others claim to read a lot, and thus obtain an escape through the imagination or the satisfaction of a thirst for knowledge. Still others maintain erotic epistolary relationships with a partner, as a way of living vicariously through the lack of sexual relations. In this case, words embody the power to replace the closeness of human beings.

The women say the same thing as the men about the impossibility of compensating for sexual relations. Marseille expresses the view that "a sexual relationship with someone you love has no possible substitute". Even if the absence of sexual relations causes a *drop in energy* and a feeling of *profound loneliness*, it's more the emotional dimension that women seek to compensate for. So for those lucky enough to have regular visits to the visiting room, even if sexual excitement is not excluded, satisfaction and serenity come mainly from the feeling of remaining essential to a spouse they love.

In any case, when the libido remains awake, the management of frustrated sexual desires remains a daily obsession to contain unfulfilled desires, which can only be alleviated by an escape involving an expenditure of energy. In

---

52. Tom is 37, incarcerated at the œrmingen detention center.

any case, the need to compensate for the deprivation of sexual relations is proportional to the intensity of the sexual needs to be compensated. Some people find it easy to forget, doing everything in their power not to think about sex. Others, provided they have a partner on the outside, manage to sublimate their desire through writing, epistolary correspondence and telephone calls. In conclusion, as Jacques Lesage de La Haye points out, there is no possible compensation: "The sexual need is never fulfilled; the deprivation of sexual relations is, in fact, a time bomb."[53]

Body integrity, sport and other narcissistic reappropriations

The deprivation of sexual relations is not without influence on the self-image that needs to be restored, following the maxim: "To please oneself is already to please someone". As a result, a form of libidinal compensation is put in place through sporting activities, particularly weight training. Almost all detention centers are equipped with sports facilities, fields and halls, and qualified sports instructors, often recruited from the ranks of prison guards. Team sports have the advantage of strengthening the cohesion within inmate teams, and offering challenges that provide perspectives in a period of detention in which the days follow one another tirelessly. The benefits of bodybuilding are particularly relevant to sexual issues. Body sculpting is a way of reappropriating oneself by maintaining one's own body, with the aim of preserving an integrity perceived as a form of resistance to the hold of the prison institution.

The narcissistic dimension involved in working on one's body in order to appreciate it, compensates in part for the narcissistic image usually projected by sexual partners when seduction and sexuality are possible. Since inmates no longer have the opportunity to please in a relationship with otherness, the aim is to please oneself in a relationship

---

53. Interview conducted in Paris in 2005.

with one's own singularity in the form of autoeroticism, which is not necessarily genital in nature. Bodybuilding does not compensate for libidinal impulses in their pleasure dimension, nor in the satisfaction of the senses aroused during a sexual relationship. As with other sporting activities, it's more a question of compensating for the ancillary contributions of sexuality, and repairing a body image degraded day after day by deprivation and the very principle of imprisonment. Dominique Lhuilier *et al.* explain this by referring to the "extreme dependence on the satisfaction of the most essential needs"[54].

The pride that male prisoners can take in their physical appearance and the prowess they are able to display, helps *reassure* a virility weakened by numerous deprivations, submission to authority and the absence of opportunities for seduction. Bodybuilding is an investment in effort and time, enabling those who practice it to reinvest their sense of power. This practice is not limited to the satisfaction of self-image in a one-to-one mirror relationship. It also includes the existence of the other's gaze in a game of exhibition of this bodily envelope, which valorizes, in proportion to the envy it arouses through the gaze in the changing rooms or in the shower. It's the strategic creation of a natural armour to defend against the physical and mental domination of other inmates. It's also the evocation of the place that some want to take, that others want to impose, underlining the primordial issue of self-evaluation by otherness. The pleasure derived from this exhibition is more or less assumed, insofar as it induces the recognition by men that the gaze of other men brings benefits comparable to the gaze of women. This relationship of seduction appears as a *passive homosexuality* that does not correspond to the desire for the body of another of the same sex as oneself, but to the enjoyment of pleasing this *other self*, in the

---

54. Veil (Claude) et Lhuilier (Dominique), (sous la direction de), *La Prison en changement*, Ramonville Saint-Agne, Érès, coll. "Trajet", 2000, p. 209.

elaboration of a mirror relationship that does not necessarily exclude sexual desire, but does not consciously envisage it as an essential goal.

Tattooing is also a technique used to sublimate a form of libido on the skin, through ornamental expression. Tattooing makes the body exist as a support to be displayed. It restores a function to a body that is no longer looked at, to a skin that is no longer caressed. At the heart of a normalizing institution, it also allows individuals to be singled out. Used since time immemorial in prisons and jails, tattoos are a way of imposing power. They force the gaze of others on visual representation, but also reveal a virility deduced from the physical suffering endured as the price of the power on which the self-image is built. When men's value is no longer measured by the exhibition of their conquests, when power is no longer reflected by the women who are made to come, when the body is no more than flesh that is filled with bad food, emptied under mediocre hygiene conditions, and maintained in showers that deny intimacy, the challenge is to rediscover a capacity to *be excited* by the *illusion of being exciting*. There's this search for the over-valuing of a being, devalued by the deprivation of sexual relations and humiliated by imprisonment. It's about maintaining a body that remains as the last possession, the one that only death, with its depersonalized power, can seize. The body is more than a carnal envelope, since it becomes the representative of the intimate being, of the whole existence, day after day emptied of emotions and events.

The Greek myth of Narcissus[55] is organized around the face, which represents the entire body: "Without suspecting it, he desires himself,

---

55. Cursed by a young man whose love he refuses, also refusing that of the nymphEcho, the young Narcissus, meets his image in a fountain, falls in love with her and dies because he can't reach her. This fable is told by Conon, Pausanias, Philostratus and Ovid in *The Metamorphoses*, Book III.

he is the lover and the object. What does he see? He doesn't know, but what he sees consumes him; the same error that deceives his eyes excites them."[56] As the years go by, sexuality in prison no longer necessarily implies a relationship with the other, but encourages the development of self-centered mental constructs. The de-socialization experienced as a consequence of confinement is also related to this sexual issue, which isolates the individual from the group, to the point of making him or her an entity independent of any system. Sexual death and social death are intimately linked, like Narcissus becoming one with the object of otherness: "I don't have long to live, I'm dying in my prime. Death is not cruel to me, for it relieves me of my pains; I wish this object of my tenderness had a longer existence, but, united by the heart, we die breathing the same sigh."[57]

Strengths and limits of solo practices

> "Masturbation is a way of pleasuring myself with someone I love."
> (Woody Allen)

In the minds of prisoners, masturbation is not a *de facto part* of sexuality. It's an ancillary practice, considered initiatory in adolescence, then incidental in adulthood. The prison administration also draws a distinction between sexuality involving the mixing of bodies, and masturbatory activities likely to be surprised on a daily basis by the use of the eyepiece. In one case, the scene is one of indecent exposure, justifying the prohibition of sexual relations. In the other case, we are faced with a situation that 18th and 19th century criminal lawyers have long tried to combat, like an addiction that can be continually

---

56. Ovid, *Les Métamorphoses*, Paris, Les Belles Lettres, 1985, book II, p. 87.
57. *Ibid.*

satisfied[58], but with less obsession than the eradication of homosexual behavior. Today's prison administration tolerates masturbation, which it cannot control, and even encourages it through the use of pornography.

Regression and guilt in masturbation

"That unnatural practice by which persons of either sex may defile their bodies, without the assistance of others. Abandoning themselves to their filthy imagination, they strive to imitate and procure for themselves the sensation which God has seen fit to accompany the carnal commerce of both sexes for the perpetuation of our species."[59]

It is symptomatic to note that recounting masturbatory practices has always seemed more difficult than evoking sexual practices as a couple. An obvious sense of modesty has mostly governed discourse on masturbation. While the evocation of fellatio, sodomy and other sexual practices was unrestricted, masturbation in prison was evoked by metaphorical expressions, more or less ironic but nonetheless meaningful, such as Alfred's: "We wash dirty laundry by hand", or Max's: "I take myself in hand." The feeling of regression seems to be the driving force behind the guilt surrounding masturbation in detention. It's both the memory of adolescent guilt linked to a sexual practice that is sometimes forbidden. It's also a regression, a reminder of the offence committed. Finally, it's the guilt that surrounds the shame of feeling diminished to the point of being deprived of otherness, of being reduced to arousing no one and arousing only oneself. In the context of solitary pleasure, sexual guilt is not shared. In sexual relations, however, guilt is mitigated by the partners' combined desire to contribute to a shared and hypothetically simultaneous enjoyment, in a simulacrum of the reproductive act.

---

58. LAQUEUR (Thomas), *Le Sexe en solitaire*, translated from English by Pierre-Emmanuel Dauzat, Paris, Gallimard, 2005, p. 261.
59. Author unknown, *in* LAQUEUR (Thomas), *op. cit.* p. 29.

Women, on the other hand, report little or no use of masturbation. Whether they consider the adolescent period or the deprivation of sexual relations, solitary sexuality appears for the most part as a solution rejected as unsuitable for compensating for the lack of intimate relations. Women's discourse most often attests to an indispensable association between affection or admiration on the one hand, and sexual excitement on the other. Sexuality is experienced as a need to touch, to cherish, a whole set of behaviors that place pleasure at the level of the feeling of being two, of existing for the other, more than at the level of the excitation of a specific erogenous zone. Eight out of the eleven women we met said they had never tried masturbation, while Lily explained that she masturbates "when [her] body feels like it", and Beatrice admitted to having masturbated "every night before bed" for a long time.

Memories of the first masturbation are still hazy. It seems difficult to pinpoint the exact age at which the first practices began. Responses often attest to a friendly sharing of *pleasure recipes*, as elegantly expressed: "I learned by word of mouth." Among younger inmates, it seems that the very existence of masturbation has always been known, the practice taking hold from the time pornographic films became commonplace. The feeling of regression is diffuse and can be interpreted in the discourse of all inmates. The ability to conjugate one's body with that of a partner is a prerequisite for self-esteem as an adult being. Sexual relations are free pleasures authorized by the evolution of a body that naturally transforms to the point of allowing what childhood did not authorize. The deprivation of sexual relations is experienced as the taking hostage of an adult prerogative on which the identity of the virile man is built. Man is powerful because of his ability to seduce, dominate and penetrate. When this prerogative is taken away from him, he regresses to the status of an adolescent, a pre-adult, deprived of the possibility of using his phallus, understood as a sexual toy signifying strength and power. Incarceration means regression to a de facto devirilish school status. Prison masturbation reminds inmates of the sexual practices of hostels and boarding schools. There's a sense of "back to square one" in this sensation, underlining the deprivation of otherness in detention. Rodrigue confides, "With masturbation, I feel like I'm regressing, and the worst thing is that it's not even really sexuality!" In adolescence, many accounts evoked shared masturbations, experienced as moments when men measured their attributes in reference to their power. From these episodes, men retain a memory that dictates their hierarchical place in the male gender community. Detention makes no mistake when it reconstitutes, in a monosexual universe, this house-of-men in which social bonds are built on a perpetual evaluation of men amongst themselves. This need gives rise to relationships of violence and domination, forcing all inmates to engage in potentially aggressive behavior, if only to defend themselves.

At all times, like hiding children, inmates know that male or female guards can open the eyepiece[60] and monitor sexual games inside the cells. In overcrowded prisons, intimacy is shared with fellow inmates during masturbation, which accompanies the religious silence of the pornographic film. Some reconstitute precarious intimacy by hanging up sheets.

Guilt about masturbation is also built around other parameters, notably religious. The moral condemnation of masturbation can be found in the Bible[61]. And yet, until the 18th century, masturbation was

---

60. During the night, the guards are not allowed to enter the cells. However, they do make rounds, for example, when a pornographic film is being shown on television. The perverse behavior of prison guards, often criticized by inmates, is not the fault of the corporation as a whole. However, there are exceptions, enough to darken a general reputation and penetrate the discourse of inmates, whatever the establishments frequented.
61. Onan died for working against procreation. "Book of Genesis, chapter XXXVIII, verses 8-10, *La Bible de Jérusalem*, Paris, Desclée de Brouwer, 1975, p. 60.

viewed with indulgence compared to other, far more serious sins of the flesh, such as coitus outside marriage or homosexuality. Several inmate converts explained that they were now trying to *do penance* by no longer committing the *sin of masturbation*, understood as an unnatural act. This is the case of Saul, a recent convert: "Today, I'm getting closer to religion, so I haven't been masturbating for three months. It's a bit hard, but I try not to think about it too much. Still, sex is very important to me, giving pleasure to women so that I can get pleasure myself, that's really the main thing."

Historically, masturbation has also been seen as a detour of reproductive capacities, for the purposes of solitary pleasure, reputed to be selfish, with the consequence of directing life drives towards individual satisfaction, in defiance of otherness[62]. Numerous authors have contributed to making masturbation a sinful and perverse practice, articulating arguments that are today described as fanciful. Tissot was undoubtedly the most virulent, elevating masturbation to the level of a disease in *Onania*[63]. Rousseau[64] was also a scourge of masturbatory practices, which he considered a "solitary vice of the imagination and fantasy" in *Les Confessions*, and a "cause of the collapse of the educational project" in *Émile*[65]. In a reversal of the guilt principle, in nineteenth-century moralist society, rather than blaming inhumane conditions of incarceration, inmates' ills were regularly blamed on solitary sexual practices: "Young and old, they indulge in it [masturbation and pederasty, [*nda*]

---

62. Laqueur (Thomas), *op. cit.* p. 142.
63. Tissot (Samuel Auguste André David), Clément (Emmanuel) (scientific editor), *De l'onanisme*, revu et mis à jour, Paris, publisher unknown, 1877.
64. "[...] to dispose, as it were, at their pleasure, of the whole sex, and to make the beauty that tempts them serve their pleasures, without needing to obtain her confession", "Les Confessions III", in *œuvres complètes*, Paris, Le Seuil, 1967, vol. I, p. 161.
65. Rousseau (Jean-Jacques), "Émile", in *œuvres complètes*, Paris, Gallimard, coll. "Bibliothèque de la Pléiade", 1990.

with such excess, that it is to this more than to misery, to sorrow, that the prison doctors of the Seine department whom I have consulted, attribute the frequency of pulmonary phthisis, stomach pulls, muscular weakness, debilitation of sight and intellectual faculties."[66]

From the time of Freud onwards, masturbation began to be seen as a sexual practice enabling the discovery of the body and of pleasure, in the manner of an initiatory discovery of what *true sexuality* represents. The return to this residual form of sexuality in detention is experienced as a measure of exclusion. In sexual symbolism, it represents cellular confinement, in which vital functions are maintained, while the sense of existence represented by conjugation with otherness is amputated by the punishment.

From the gradual erasure of otherness to autoeroticism

Because the lack of pleasure in the encounter with the other becomes haunting, because the daily routine of *long sentences* is repetitive, taste-less, lacking in desire and horizon, masturbatory practices are appre-hended as a means of calming, sleeping and soothing unsatisfied sexual impulses. For most inmates, the construction of the libido is limited to autoeroticism and wandering in a pre-constructed virtuality, in which the subject is no longer a *desirer* but *a consumer*, with an over-solici-tation that, like Léon, can go up to ten or twelve times a day: "Even the doctor recognized that I had great needs, so I shouldn't hesitate. In solitary confinement, I can masturbate up to twelve times a day. It's a medical prescription!"

Prisoners placed in solitary confinement or in the disciplinary section are deprived of everything. With the exception of a daily walk, where

---

66. O'Brien (Patricia), *Correction ou châtiment*, Paris, PUF, coll. "Les Chemins de l'his-toire", 1988, p. 106.

they are protected from any encounters, their only activities are reading and watching television. Masturbation then becomes a worn-out and abused practice, sometimes even leading to injury. Over time, this absence of otherness gradually turns masturbation into a form of autoeroticism, in which the imagination of the other's body becomes no more than a secondary accessory to obtaining pleasure.

By dint of forgetting this other, often fantasized as faceless and nameless, we want to please ourselves, because the surrounding world of the prison population is reduced to the solitude of a cell, late at night, and to the uniqueness of a body that remains the last possession of the dispossessed. In the narcissistic relationship, the other can only be seen as another self, and therefore of the same sex. By dint of satisfying visual arousal only with the attributes of a body that is caressed with hands that we end up attributing to another self, the gender reference remains unique, and heterosexual eroticism is deconstructed in favor of a solitary eroticism that is sometimes homosexual, sometimes excluding the other to the point of making conjugal reunion illusory upon liberation. In all cases, *duration is* an essential factor in assessing the after-effects of a sexuality maintained in solitude.

Having consummated sexuality in defiance of Saint Augustine's conception[67], the rediscovery of conjugal closeness at liberation cannot be imagined without a bump in the road. The challenge will be to restore a place for otherness and, above all, to find a place for one's own singularity, from an erotic point of view, within the framework of a relationship for two. Integrating the existence of the other when plea-

---

67. For Saint Augustine, sexuality is understood as a "conjugal duty", which he calls "conjugal charity". According to this concept, "no one owns his own body, but each one disposes of the other's". The exclusive consideration of one's own body in masturbation constitutes, by the same token, the negation of the other's body.

sure and the organ mechanism have been operating in a *closed circuit* for many years requires personal re-education. Stories of failure and multiple anguish abound in the literature of ex-convicts' testimonials: "Not only have I gone twelve years without making love, but I'm also impotent. I can't make up for lost time. [...] I just have to die. Prison makes inaffective monsters, hybrids or mutants, incapable of adapting to the world of human relationships."[68]

Organ mechanics instead of desire

Masturbation serves to extinguish tensions that have two main origins. On the one hand, the frustration of sexual desires, and on the other, anxieties born of a feeling of castration. In addition to the rarely mentioned search for pleasure, masturbation serves to check the survival of the sexual organs, especially in the case of men for whom sexual deprivation and the constraints of confinement are often equated with a progressive, throbbing and sometimes fatal loss of virility. In prison, *long-sentenced* men are faced with the worry of seeing their ability to "get it up" fade away. Bruno Bettelheim noted similar elements in relation to concentration camp confinement: "Almost all the prisoners were afraid of becoming impotent, and anxiety drove them to check their virility. They could only choose between homosexuality or masturbation. [...] Nevertheless, given their upbringing and adult standards, each of these expedients constituted a regression to adolescent behavior that aggravated their sense of guilt."[69] Masturbation is experienced as a sample, an *ersatz that makes it* possible to survive deprivation, a "spare wheel" enabling survival, not so much of sexual desires, but more of organ functioning, and the evacuation of tensions born of the frustration of unfulfilled impulses.

---

68. Lesage de La Haye (Jacques), *L'Homme de métal*, Paris, Existences, 1995, p. 49.
69. Bettelheim (Bruno), *The Conscious Heart. Comment garder son autonomie et parvenir à l'accomplissement de soi dans une civilisation de masse*, Paris, Robert Laffont, coll. "Réponses", 1972, p. 222.

One warden explains that the absence of sexual relations eventually leads to abdominal pain, which can only be alleviated by masturbation. This is known as the "ouille-ouille syndrome"[70], which seems to be familiar to individuals interrupting intense sexual activity on the outside through incarceration. Men fear that a prolonged absence of ejaculation will lead to irreversible impotence, which would prove to be an additional stigma of incarceration, in this case mutilation through progressive castration. Consequently, masturbatory practices obey an economy of managing gains and anticipating losses. This is also what reassures paranoid ideas about the use of bromide[71] in prison, as expressed by Jason, an inmate at Saint-Mihiel: "When I jerk off and ejaculate, it's a relief to know that it still works. For a while, I was afraid of losing my sexuality. I thought maybe there was something hidden in the food. There are a lot of rumors about that. So I masturbated to reassure myself."

When it comes to sexual practice, it's not so much know-how that is forgotten, but rather self-confidence, which erodes with the weight of years. The length of a prisoner's sentence is a "desert crossing", during which they forget what it means to confront their individuality with the appreciation of others. The feeling of regression generates anxieties that medical teams are charged with curbing. Dr. Acker, a doctor at the Maison d'arrêt de la Santé, explains[72] that sexual anxiety is added to the sum total of anxieties concerning the couple on release. And even if it

---

70. This is how the physical pain of not having sex seems to be described. The supervisor describes the sensation as "headache-inducing testicular tension". In his opinion, masturbation-stimulating pornography is the ideal way to remedy the "ouchiness".
71. Bromide (potassium bromide) is a chemical substance with sedative effects, long used to calm the sexual ardor of male and female prisoners, as well as military personnel. See BOUCARD (Robert), *Les Dessous des prisons de femmes*, Paris, Éditions de France, 1930, p. 80. Many rumors continue to circulate about its contemporary use.
72. Interview conducted in Paris in September 2005.

turns out that, during the interviews, the inmates were rather optimistic about resuming a couple's life on release, Jacques Lesage de La Haye points out that sexual problems often appear as if by surprise and, as a result, regularly alter the reintegration process, without this apprehension ever being concretely envisaged during the years of detention.

The reputation of the ever-powerful man feeds a taboo among males, who find it difficult to express their libido problems to their release. And yet, after decades without a partner, intimate reunion becomes a source of stress that can lead to failure. Rodrigue, an inmate at Val-de-Reuil, explains that he was apprehensive about resuming his sex life the first time he went out on leave after six years in prison. He feared he'd become a premature ejaculator. In the end, the surprise effect of a friend's *generosity* towards an *inmate in need*, combined with the disinhibition of alcohol, enabled him to serenely resume sexual relations. Daniel Welzer-Lang *et al.* have also noted the sexual problems that are bound to arise on release from *long sentences*, leading to "various disorders in terms of sexual relations and social identity. [...] Premature ejaculation and impotence are regularly mentioned."[73] To mitigate the disruptive effect of detention, the furlough system is beneficial in more ways than one. As far as sexuality is concerned, it allows us to re-experience sexual relations under temporary conditions, like a dress rehearsal. If problems arise, the psychological support offered on return to prison can sometimes help to ease the situation and open up a dialogue that would be more difficult to establish on release.

---

73. WELZER-LANG (Daniel), FAURE (Michaël), MATHIEU (Lilian), *Sexualités et violences en prison*, Lyon, OIP/Aléas, 1996, p. 93.

The limits of exclusively genital sexuality

> "If woman is reduced to a hole, if making love is nothing more than
> the piston-and-breech action of X-rated films, sex is the nothingness
> of sensation where death looms. It's the void, the abyss"[74].

This sexuality, constantly divided between impossible seduction on the one hand, and the satisfaction of a solitary orgasm on the other, is proving to be destabilizing in the development of relationships with others. Masturbation, understood as an exclusive sexual practice, remains what Sther, an inmate at Val-de-Reuil, defines as "the poor man's pittance", both inside and out. This state of poverty in the latitude left to sexuality in prison is experienced as a humiliation. Franck calls it "a diversion, a sexual release that isn't even an accomplishment". Finding himself alone every evening in front of pornographic virtuality, or psychologically mourning the loss of a libido that the body recalls, is a metaphor for the deprivation imposed by incarceration. In this total dispossession organized by the institution, only the possibility of an orgasm can preserve an inalienable sense of self-appropriation.

Yet when practiced in this way, sexuality loses the fusional capacities that make it so reassuring. What remains is the gaping absence of all those gestures that surround pleasure, that precede or follow it. The mortifying aspects are due to the absence of caresses, kisses, the closeness of skins and bodies, all the satisfaction of the senses that reminds us that we exist because the other exists and recognizes us as existing. Masturbation doesn't cure the feeling of loneliness that is omnipresent in *long sentences*. Finally, in prison, thinking about one's own existence without thinking about that of others is a more dangerous impasse

---

74. GONIN (Daniel), *La Santé incarcérée*, Paris, L'Archipel, 1991, p. 171.

than individualism and any form of forgetfulness of others, their rights and possessions. The deprivation of sexual relations is thus perceived as the antechamber of death, a premature old age, which would affect a population that is still young and in demand.

The material reconstitution of otherness

> "Desire is the wish to consume, to drink, to devour, to ingest, then to digest - to annihilate. It requires no other prompter than the presence of otherness."[75]

In the same way that solitary masturbation wearies the inmates, they gradually try to reconstruct sexual practices that will rekindle desire, mixing a panoply of substitutes. New practices are tried out, multiple scenarios are invented, accessories are cobbled together. Survival and the satisfaction of the libido call for a wealth of adaptations, sometimes going as far as substitutive zoophilic practices[76], which would not fail to shock outside society, which imagines, in a Manichean conception, that such excesses only exist in prison. Here again, the institution doesn't invent anything. What exists in prison already exists outside, albeit in different proportions, and certainly for less compelling reasons. Monosexual confinement and the prohibition of sexual relations lead to a paucity of objects of excitement and changes in desire: "[...] Some inmates peel the stamps off letters they receive from their wives or girl-

---

75. BAUMAN (Zygmunt), *L'Amour liquide. De la fragilité des liens entre les hommes*, Rodez, Le Rouergue/Chambon, 2004, p. 19.
76. Although rare, cases of zoophilia are frequently recounted in the testimonies of former inmates. For example: "On several occasions, we have been told of scenes of collective sodomy involving cats, of which there are many in certain prisons such as Fresnes and Marseille. Some of these animals meet a rather sad end, caught by inmates who know how to put them in confidence, the cats are often killed after having been sodomized and having undergone a certain number of torments, the least severe of which appears to be the plucking out of their eyes", MONNEREAU (Alain), *La Castration pénitentiaire. Droit à la sexualité pour les personnes incarcérées*, Paris, Lumière et Justice, 1986, p. 45.

friends and run their own tongues over them, knowing that the loved one has run his or hers over them. [...] In this way, it has been reported to us that prisoners masturbate and cum between two cakes that they will offer to their lover."[77]

To alleviate the suffering inflicted by the growing lack, the inmates piece together, like a jigsaw puzzle, the components of the sexuality that is so lacking. They try to satisfy their senses with the meager possessions allowed in detention. The aim is to rediscover touch, smell or the sensation of an entire organ. Recipes that have long been tried and tested include reconstituting a woman's vagina using a washcloth filled with hot pasta, or penetrating a mattress pierced with a carefully designed orifice. Because these practices don't always make you proud, Kappa refers to them modestly, finding it easier to talk about others than about himself: "I know quite a few people who reconstruct vaginas of all kinds." Marcus, who has accumulated incarcerations in several different countries, recalls "attempts to penetrate hot chickens... and cats too!"

Sometimes, it's a more elaborate re-enactment, allowing the sensations of a body around sex to be rediscovered: "He rolls up a blanket with a wet plastic bag, using the 'baisette' method [...] Then he slips the bottom of the blanket into the underwear. This forces him to pull the underwear apart to penetrate the bag, which is flooded with saliva or warm oil. Thoroughly aroused, he comes to imagine that he's sleeping with his wife without undressing her completely, and sinks into lightning orgasms."[78]

---

77. *Ibid*, p. 46.
78. LESAGE DE LA HAYE (Jacques), *La Guillotine du sexe. La vie affective et sexuelle des prisonniers*, Paris, L'Atelier/Éditions Ouvrières, 1998, p. 192.

In one sense or another, men strive to recreate the sensation of penetration, believing that coitus is indissociable from sexuality, involving for the most part the interweaving of two bodies, which, for the duration of the practice, make us forget the sense of existential solitude that frightens, anguishes and makes us dizzy. In Caen, Garouda recalls the DIY projects that everyone organizes, with the pseudo-complicity of the administration, which struggles to set limits even in the pottery workshop: "I made a dildo with a wooden skittle, and I cover it with a condom so as not to hurt myself. [...] One guy was making dildos for everyone in the pottery workshop. Eventually, the supervisors asked him to stop." These practices may be the continuation of a sexuality that predates incarceration. For some, it's despair combined with the length of long sentences that leads to the development of behaviors and stagings, to the credit of a feeling of degradation. Others finally fuel their excitement with exhibitionist behavior, which they express in the shower or in front of windows: "Prison forbids him to make love. He found a way to do it anyway. If you can call it that... He gets naked, climbs onto the windowsill and masturbates for his friend's benefit."[79] These narratives are reminiscent of Arnould Galopin's descriptions in the nineteenth century[80], when he reported on the development of sexual vices in the difficult daily lives of incarcerated women.

"For prisons kill souls, crumble consciences. Women who have suffered captivity leave their cells enraged and evil. [...] By wanting

---

79. *Ibid*, p. 167.

80. Arnould Galopin's work, based on biftons (correspondence between women in prison), has been widely criticized in terms of authenticity. Nevertheless, the description of women's prisons at the end of the 19th and beginning of the 20th centuries speaks volumes about the conditions of incarceration at the time, and about the rupture between inside and outside that can still be found today in the current system of incarceration. See ARTIÈRES (Philippe) and LAÉ (Jean-François), *Lettres perdues. Écriture, amour et solitude, xixe-xxe siècle*, Paris, Hachette Littératures, 2003, p. 180.

to punish these unfortunate women, society has inflicted a punishment on itself, for as long as it is unable to proportion the punishment to the crime or misdemeanor, it will always create rebels, the 'entrenched' of vice, with whom it will be forced to engage in a merciless struggle"[81].

Inaccessible objects of desire

In terms of desire, the contingencies of confinement constitute a disconnect between the reality outside and the experience inside. Excitement mechanisms have to be rebuilt on the basis of a virtuality that fuels desire in the context of missing otherness. By dint of their absence from monosexual detention, women become, for men, subjects of imagination and desire, according to a Manichean categorization. Images replace sight and touch. Memories of the past are moments continually reapprehended in the present. Excitement in detention resembles the fragile recomposition of a *jigsaw puzzle*, from which prisoners will attempt to maintain the existence of desire in the context of a chaotic and insufficient sex life. In terms of desire, but also of social recognition of the other gender, monosexual confinement poses the problem of the survival of the memory of *who the other is*. This is all the more true given that in prison, social gender roles are turned upside down: male prisoners are at the mercy of the women on whom they depend. They are openly in a position of expectation and demand. They are no longer the protectors, but rather the ones who need attention, empathy and tenderness. This regression, imposed by detention, turns them into children in waiting, while the women take on a maternal role.

---

81. GALOPIN (Arnould), *Les Enracinées*, Paris, Fayard, 1902, p. 16.

The women the inmates talk about are sometimes imaginary. Some of them remain attached to the spouse they left at the institution's door. Others have potential conquests recommended to them, and initiate relationships through letter-writing and photo-sending, which have only the speed of desire transactions to envy *internet dating*. However, for the vast majority of long-sentence prisoners, the celibacy imposed by monosexual confinement is a reality that lasts until it becomes an exclusive, timeless *way of being*.

In prison, encounters with the opposite sex are limited to female warders, nurses and social workers. The setback caused by the inability to meet the opposite sex fuels men's descriptive discourses of "women we love" and "women we fuck". This categorization is not exclusive to closeted men. However, the absence of women reinforces this imaginary, divided conception. At a distance from the reality of impossible seduction, the feeling of castrated virility is compensated for by an authoritarian judgment that gains in importance during imprisonment. The descriptions underpin a machismo exacerbated by the feeling of a degraded virility. The vision of women is binary and built around relationships to sexuality. In both cases, categorization appears to be a masculine prerogative of the man who decides, judges, uses as he pleases and condemns. Karim, an inmate at Val-de-Reuil, says of sexual discussions: "There's a taboo about the woman you're with, the one you love. But mistresses, yes, we can talk about them, and even tell everything."

Female wives and breeders

There are women you marry and flaunt. These encounters have a narcissistic dimension: they are the image of what men feel *they officially deserve*. These are also the women with whom reproduction is conceivable or already a reality. These women's bodies are worthy enough to bear their personal offspring. The relationship is based on a form of possession. The man is protective in exchange for the admiration he must arouse. These women are respected by men, according to criteria they alone define. They represent the idealized continuity of the mother in adult life, the mother the inmates have had, or the one they have fantasized about, the one who will protect their offspring, and the one they protect as a male protects his offspring. They are objects of affection before they are objects of pleasure. The expression of a need for domination is compensated for by the demand for respect, with conditions imposed in an authoritarian manner of course, but auguring serenity when consent is equitable. These are women to whom men recognize the possibility of female sexual pleasure, which must nevertheless remain confined to a sexuality conditional on emotional commitment.

It's symptomatic to note that the young inmates (under 26), although belonging to the robbers and kingpins, positioned their mother as the essential woman, taking precedence over all others. These evocations express a dichotomy between a desire to appear virile and powerful, and the conscious or unconscious feeling of remaining dependent on an adult mother like a child who has not grown up. This confusion is reflected, for example, in the speech of Ryan, seducer and glutton for the pleasures of the flesh, who, when asked, "Are you in love right now?" thinks for a moment, then replies, "Yes, with my mother, she's 54, but she's the best!"

Preferably, this idealized woman must be a virgin, and above all, faithful. Zizou explains: "You can't do cunnilingus to just anyone. It's only possible with a girl who hasn't been used several times. Ideally, I'd like to find a virgin. I want to be the first and only one. It's also a question of hygiene and respect." Unsurprisingly, from the male point of view, the rules of fidelity are considered indisputable for women and negotiable for men. The price of exclusivity, determined by an unspoken contract, lies in the man's gift of his ability to defend himself on the one hand, and of reproductive semen on the other. However, these women are not idealized as princesses to whom men would cede everything. The seduction involved is a temporal, emotional and material investment to establish a feeling of possession. In their rigidity, these discourses attest to the distortion that the duration of celibacy ultimately brings about among long-sentenced prisoners. It's not so much a question of asserting that prison generates macho conceptions, but rather of concluding that a radically binary conception is exacerbated, feeding on shortcomings, a feeling of eroded virility and a lack of understanding of a changing society, in which the female gender no doubt does not express the same expectations today as it did yesterday.

Female sex objects: clean and dirty

They are "the ones we fuck and despise". Their description speaks volumes about the gender hierarchy, exacerbated in detention to enhance a degraded and weakened sense of power. These women are commodified for the satisfaction of pleasure and *ego*. They are so-called *"easy* women", whom men pretend to "pass off" to their buddies, as objects at the service of male pleasure, and whose consent alone is guaranteed by the pleasure men pretend to give them. They are seen as people who have already been soiled by the levity of their previous sexual adventures, which dishonors them once and for all. It's therefore possible to indulge every sexual fantasy with them. Ryan declares that he enjoys sodomizing a girl, but not just any girl: "I'm not going to sodomize a girl I love, I have too much respect for her. Besides, how can you imagine my wife kissing my son if she's sucked me off first? It's disgusting!"

There is no investment in these women. The notion of respect doesn't exist, since the sexuality practiced with them is devoid of any reproductive vocation or sentimental involvement. With these *women of ill repute,* men allow themselves to defy the laws of hygiene: dirtiness is possible, since dirtiness pre-exists the encounter. The men allow themselves to degrade them, since they themselves have previously allowed themselves to be degraded in the context of unbridled sexuality, real or imagined.

Although this concept is mainly confined to young inmates, it nonetheless testifies to an *intramural* evolution in the consideration of rapists of women. Traditionally, pointers were mainly adult rapists. Today, paedophilia is the most productive illegalism in terms of incarceration[82]. This is also the analysis of Gayle S. Rubin when he writes: "For more than a century, no strategy for arousing sexual hysteria has worked as well as the call to protect children."[83] In the discourse of prisoners, the cursor of the unacceptable today tends to move to the side of child abusers. The new generation of inmates is tending to modify their assessment of the rape of adult women, through a blurred and indecisive recognition of the notion of consent, particularly when evoking the phenomenon of *tournantes*. We are witnessing a reclassification of the notion of victim. The women abused during these collective practices are precisely those objects with whom all *sexual fantasies are* conceivable, as soon as, as Tom points out, a detail in their physical appearance prompts them to envisage them: "With women, it's sometimes ambiguous, there are women who can take advantage of it and then deny consent. But with a child, it's always guilty. But with a 16-year-old girl, sometimes she provokes, she doesn't want to realize that we like to watch. At school, it's not acceptable to dress short, even at clubs!

Jason describes male/female relations as an unequal balance of power, thwarted by legal provisions in favor of women, and underpinned by

---

82. Sexual delinquency accounts for 18.8% of convicts in prison, i.e. 8,250 men and 160 women. See TOURNIER (Pierre V.), *op. cit.* in "Lettre d'information sur les questions pénales", no. 54, September 10, 2007.
83. RUBIN (Gayle S.), *Penser le sexe. Pour une théorie radicale de la politique de la sexualité*, Epel, Paris, 2001, p. 72.

potentially contradictory interests. The assessment of consent remains, in the discourse of male prisoners, a male prerogative: "It depends how it goes, whether it's a girlfriend we know or not. Girls are quick to complain now. [...] In a couple there's never rape, unless there's violence, physical coercion." As for Ryan, he suggests putting rapists in prison for life and speaks out in favor of capital punishment for pedophiles, while at the same time, this is how he recounts his experience of tournantes: "Among the women I've fucked, there are twenty chicks I've respected, fifty whores and ten sluts. We did some tournantes, some sort of partouses. Once, with some buddies, there were ten of us on one chick. She consented."

This conception of women is based on the recognition that female pleasure is equivalent to male pleasure. Except that the inmates reproach them for having chosen pleasure and freedom at the cost of an indelible reputation that does not deserve respect. This dishonorable choice is a *dirty* choice. Prisoners often combine desire and hygiene. *Cleanliness* reassures the integrity of the body, which remains the only residual possession in detention. Confinement is experienced as soiling. Noises, smells and waste are combined with the collective. Alfred complains: "You feel dirty here, even when you're clean. The totalizing aspect of the prison ends up making us fear the disappearance of distinctive boundaries between the self and others, notably because of all the places we have to share, the individuals who use the same space, this community densified into a few hundred square meters. Zizou, for example, is obsessed with a notion of hygiene that determines right and wrong. This is the main motivation behind his prohibitions. Moreover, although he claims to be tolerant, he believes that homosexuality is not clean. For him, sexuality in prison is unthinkable because of the lack of hygiene.

The limits of co-education or the caste hierarchy

Seducing a female warder is something that inmates can envisage, and even often attempt, even if they recognize that this seduction is sterile in terms of prospects, given the inescapable hierarchical distinction, dividing individuals by their membership of the inmate group as opposed to the warder group. Hierarchically, disciplinary power is held by an authority *armed with keys*, representing the symbol of power for some and freedom for others. However, in terms of desire, a measured game is organized between the inmate population and the professional actors of prison life. There's no shortage of situations in prison where intimacy is on display. Between searches, eyepiece inspections and the supervision of visiting rooms, there are numerous opportunities for inmates to confront their attitude with the gaze of women from the prison administration. A study carried out on the organization of co-education in prisons, gives the following results: "The professional gestures that pose the greatest difficulty for women working in male prisons are shower supervision (61.4%), palpation searches if they have to be carried out (57.6%), intervention in a promenade yard (51.6%) and intervention in a night cell (41%)".[84]

The presence of women is greatly appreciated. For example, Hippocampe admits: "You're gentler with a woman than with a man. It limits aggressiveness and commands respect." On the other hand, female pointers feel more judged by female supervisors, who identify with women who have been abused, or who are more shocked by acts of paedophilia. Levis, a sex offender detained at Saint-Mihiel, admits: "As long as they don't attack me on the facts of why I'm here, I let it slide... The only two who have been unpleasant with me are women"; he adds: "They know why I'm here, they've identified me. They have a

---

84. Inizan (Juliette), Deveaux (Solenne), Vêtu (Jean-Jacques), *Surveillantes en détention hommes*, Paris, T&D, Direction de l'administration pénitentiaire, 2002, p. 28.

right to know, it's the basis of a sincere relationship, and so with them, I don't stand a chance."

Generally speaking, female warders, nurses, teachers or any other female person, represent those women who are missing from the reality of detention, and who will never be replaced by the virtuality of photos or television images. It's not so much a question of sexuality to be consumed, but rather a confrontation with the opposite gender, in a relationship of seduction that's meant to be reassuring. Zizou admits: "I need to flirt, I'm a man. I miss the fact that I can't seduce anymore, so it's normal to try it here, even if it's forbidden." The fact that there are so few women for so many men is bound to arouse covetousness, most often based on illusions that each man values in himself: "I'm very charming, I like talking to women. It makes up for the lack of relationships. Sometimes I fantasize about them. Seduction happens, but it's difficult because you have to be wary of people who talk, the fellow inmates are jealous."[85]

An inmate is rarely worth the risk of a female guard risking her job for a romantic or sexual relationship. This stated certainty sends each man back to the value he represents in detention. Confinement and the deprivation of sexual relations force a necessary adjustment of male pretensions in terms of power over women. However, like many, Ryan allows himself seduction, without being fooled about the possible outcome: "We laugh with each other, but nothing will happen, because they're afraid of losing their jobs and they have what they want on the outside: they didn't wait for my zguègue!" Titi also expresses his resignation in the face of these women, whom he assumes are sexually satisfied in this outside world that exists beyond the perimeter walls:

---

85. Kappa, aged 35. Sentenced to twelve years for armed robbery, and detained at Saint-Mihiel.

"I admit there'll be nothing, that's all." Karim seduces all the women present in detention because it makes him feel good, but he knows the limits of this *forbidden and inaccessible fruit*: "You mustn't forget where I am, a female guard will never give up her salary for an inmate!" This situation is reminiscent of all the situations in which anathema is hurled when two social groups mix, contrary to the recommendations of a social order. Every society enacts and organizes relationships that are stamped with the label *unnatural*, according to a customary rule that must be respected on pain of exclusion, condemnation or denigration. Yet the power of the forbidden creates ambiguities that exacerbate desires. However, the magnitude of the ban is matched only by the suspicion it arouses in a closed universe where any notion of intimacy is illusory, and where the speed at which rumors spread is carried by the incessant gaze of all. This is also Henry's observation when he fatalistically sums up: "She's a nurse, and I'm an inmate. There's a barrier. I can't promise that she was attracted, but it felt like it. But there's the constant presence of warders and colleagues, so we're never alone. It's impossible to go all the way."

There are some who break free of this prohibition, certainly more than the rare cases that the law of silence allows to escape. But the risk is great. Failure to respect the boundary is a dishonor that underlines the prevalence of individual desires over almighty discipline. This accusation works in all gender combinations. Such unions are often ended by reason, so great is the possibility of sanction. Tony, who we met in Saint-Mihiel, recalls an affair that lasted two months: "Yes, it happened with my forewoman in Mulhouse. So we fucked in the workshops, almost every day for two months."

This was also the case for Saul with a nurse psychologist: "The relationship lasted two years, but with the constant fear of being discovered. She was 37 and I was 19. It was love at first sight. I loved her, but

110

not the way she wanted. It was the love of someone who wants her own happiness. But prison and time, and stress no doubt, destroyed my feelings. And then she risked losing her job, so I preferred to ask to be transferred to this prison." In both cases, the confession of these forbidden relationships was much more difficult than any other sexual narrative, like the revelation of the ultimate fault, the consequences of which are more painful for the women involved than for the male prisoners. It was therefore at this precise moment in the interview that the anonymity governing this investigation proved to be an indispensable condition for the discourse.

Even if the presence of women is unanimously perceived as beneficial, by the prison administration as much as by the inmates, this censorship of seductive relationships becomes suspect for male inmates. Over time, the power of the ban stigmatizes a feeling of incapacity felt by individuals who, respectively, must mourn the loss of any emotional interaction in contact with each other.

Women's masculine objects

Sexual arousal in female prisoners is more nocturnal than diurnal. It's not a sustained, artificially or mechanically generated excitement, but the resurgence of desires that arise from unconscious activity during dreams. Lily confides: "At night, you dream that you're making love and then you wake up and there's nothing... It feels weird. My subconscious is working." Sexuality responds to a desire, not a need. As there is no challenge in the exercise of sexuality, women don't feel the need to maintain practices for the sole reason of checking that their bodies are working properly, or to fuel sexual discussions that rarely exist in female detention. Nor do they feel degraded by the lack of sexual practice, although carnal deprivation is openly expressed. For the women, otherness is reassuring, to satisfy cravings for tenderness or expressions of affection, in response to feelings of loneliness. Talk of sexual pleasure is not veiled. It is, however, modestly expressed. While sexual relations mostly require an emotional investment, sexual practice is not evoked as a sentimental expression, but rather as a search for pleasure, a desire for penetration and a way of exulting in a body abandoned in detention.

At the Bapaume detention center, after banning the wearing of earrings, management has just prohibited the purchase of perfume. This measure is seen as a mutilation of femininity, and a clear abuse of the power of domination of the prison authorities, in this case formulated by a male director, anxious to prevent the male inmates of the same establishment from organizing a traffic in alcoholic substances. Myriam points out that this kind of provision, which might seem secondary, is actually the hardest thing about prison: "Here, we're deprived of everything. Now we're deprived of perfume, because some men have drunk it: they don't know what to drink! And we're not free to do our own thing. Here, we're entitled to nothing because of the men's regime." Such an arrangement lends credence to Philippe Combessie's conclusions when he explains that "the under-representation of women in prisons is detrimental to female inmates"[86].

In terms of desire, the major difference with men lies in their ability to accept the sensory lethargy of a body, without women expressing a questioning of their femininity in terms of self-esteem. Myriam distinguishes between men and women when it comes to the deprivation of sexual relations: "A man remains a man, a man needs a woman. A hole remains a hole for him. A woman goes less often than a man to get laid."

And yet, without desire and without being desired, femininity withers and fades. But instead of needing, as men do, to reassure their narcissistic

---

86. COMBESSIE (Philippe), *Sociologie de la prison*, Paris, La Découverte, coll. "Repères", 2001, p. 32.

image, it's through the search for tenderness, often between women in detention, that they manage to compensate for the absence of sexuality: "Apart from the lack of objects of seduction, what's essential to remain a woman is a loving gaze, desire [...] I try to be correct, not to have a scary face. [...] I try to be correct, not to have a scary face. [...] To be desired, that's what's missing. But here, what's the point!"[87]

In the same way as erectile dysfunction in men, the absence of sexuality and combined desire causes physiological as well as psychological transformations in women. Alain Monnereau notes: "A veritable sexual involution, reflected in the disappearance of menstruation, loss of color in the vaginal mucosa, vulval atrophy... as if a flower were closing."[88] These consequences, which each individual will have to deal with as a potential obstacle to resocialization, attest to the fact that a body that is no longer *desired or desiring*, becomes the abandoned envelope of individuals wandering in existential emptiness.

Managing excitement

Because it is deprived of otherness, sexuality in detention is limited to the horizon of the self, in sexual practices that involve memories, accessories and artificial excitements, with little possibility of identification. As the reality of arousal objects fades from memory, masturbation soon feeds on pornography. It becomes necessary to regenerate exhausted fantasies. For others, memories may suffice, and some inmates have confessed to masturbating only if an erotic dream dictates natural

---

87. Corinne Rostaing quoting Larissa, 23, from a middle-class background, sentenced to two years for theft, and incarcerated for seven months, *in* ROSTAING (Corinne), *La Relation carcérale. Identités et rapports sociaux dans les prisons de femmes*, Paris, PUF, coll. "Le Lien social", 1997, p. 269.
88. MONNEREAU (Alain), *op. cit.* p. 43.

arousal, without mechanical activation. Sexual arousal requires regular feeding of fantasies, through the satisfaction of the senses. In prison, the most easily satisfied sense is sight, so pornographic images remain the most accessible vector of arousal. Indeed, the prison administration pulls *out all the stops to ensure* that, in the alcoves of individual cells, inmates are sufficiently fed with fantasies, in order to release individual urges that we don't want to see expressed collectively in behaviors of violence, rebellion and domination.

Fluctuating libido

> "Entry into detention provokes a trauma, one of the effects of which (more or less lasting) is the "anaesthesia" of any sexual or erotic preoccupation."[89]

Prisoners were questioned about the evolution of their libido based on their legal career. This implies considering a period ranging from arrest, to conviction, to detention in a penal institution, via the status of remand prisoner waiting for long periods in overcrowded remand prisons. Libido is thus understood as a quantitative notion expressing desire and all sexual impulses. The evolution of the prevalence of this desire was analyzed through a self-assessment asked of each person, with the aim of identifying the conscious presence of desire through an analysis of sexual preoccupations in both thought and deed.

Prior to their incarceration, none of the inmates we met had imagined the issue of deprivation. Gradually, in the first few weeks of detention, the reality of sexuality in prison dawned on them, summed up in the desire for sexuality for two, only to consume it alone. Admittedly, this is not a typical prison situation. Not everyone on the outside has a partner to satisfy their desire for carnal relations. They do, however, evolve in

---

89. WELZER-LANG (Daniel), FAURE (Michaël), MATHIEU (Lilian), *op. cit.* p. 88.

a society that enables them to feed their desires, through furtive or structured encounters, and to stimulate or satisfy their senses through factual confrontation with the human race.

Men easily associate the survival of their libido with the subsistence of erections upon awakening. It's the meaning of a *desire that exists in spite of itself*, without recourse to mechanical devices. For them, it's the most convincing revelation of the integrity of their sexual functioning, both psychically and physically. Nocturnal ejaculations, non-existent or rare for most male prisoners, also represent the satisfaction of a sexuality to which the body and mind have natural, instinctive access. It's the expression of a libido that reassures, of a body that remembers, and the pleasure is all the more intense, so close is the virtuality of excitement to the reality of a sexuality that includes the other. This is how Ryan describes this particular satisfaction: "When I don't jerk off, I have a lot of polluted dreams. It's much better than masturbation. It's like I've really made love. The problem is that afterwards my sheets are dirty, and I have to take a shower before going to work. And as the water is cold in the morning, I prefer not to have to shower."[90] At the same time, nocturnal ejaculations represent a pleasure that humiliates, repulses and degrades, with the feeling of adolescent regression. The quality of sexual pleasure obtained in this way sometimes comes at the price of these paradoxes: a need that is all the more satisfying because it is unconsciously fulfilled in conditions so uncomfortable that they constitute the price of delight.

As with masturbation, the assessment of libido involves a discourse that oscillates between anxieties about loss of integrity and the search for pleasure. In both cases, it's about a feeling of life, as opposed to the

---

90. Ryan is 20 years old. He is incarcerated in Saint-Mihiel.

death anxiety metaphorized in castration anxiety, in the feeling of being reduced to nothing because neither desired nor desiring. Generally speaking, for both men and women, the intensity of the libido diminishes during the first period of incarceration.

As the years in prison pile up, talk of the movement of libido follows a *Gaussian curve*, determining a sharp fall, an intense rise and then a slow and certain fall, due to the weariness of residual prison practices. Among the factors invoked to justify these variations in libido, prisoners cite the shock of deprivation of liberty combined with the shock of the confinement that accompanies it. This new configuration of life requires an adaptation that is as risky in the overcrowding and collective cell confinement of prisons as it is conceivable in the cellular intimacy of detention centers. Multi-cell confinement makes people lose all sexual desire, unless they slip into collective homosexual practices, in which consent is often secondary. Those incarcerated for the first time often discover incarceration in the hostility of the prison, and their primary problems are more to do with safeguarding their physical integrity. The constant presence of the collective also leads to a loss of control over one's own sexuality. Particularly when erotic reference points disappear, replaced by a monosexual vision of existence. There's a dichotomy between the virtual visual acquired through pornography, and the real visual embodied by the naked bodies of people of the same sex.

Libido is also disrupted by feelings of hatred linked to conviction. It's a question of self-hatred when inmates, mainly sex offenders, evoke self-loathing and the multiple faces of guilt that imprisonment reminds them of. It's also about hatred of the institution. This is the case, for example, of Saturnin, for whom imprisonment and its trail of injustices represent a tunnel without perspective, in which nothing exists any more. Desires and prisons are often incompatible: "I don't want to mix the two worlds, which are incomparable. My life is here and I feel too much like it's got nothing to do with me. I don't want to confuse my head with what's going on outside. I don't even look at the landscape. Here I can't see far."

Depending on the reasons for the offence, the self-image is disturbed at the start of incarceration, by the public humiliation of the forthcoming trial, the discovery of the facts, and the regressive feeling of the child taken at fault by the parental hierarchy. All these elements reduce the desire to nothing. These analyses are specific to *long-sentence offenders* who discover prison and for whom, in view of the offence committed, incarceration will be a long-term process. Bruce, an inmate at Val-de-Reuil, explains that the suspension of his libido while in prison corresponds to the suspension of his life. Béa, newly married while in prison, confesses that from the point of view of desire: "Life has stopped, I'm dead but I'm going to rise again."

For women, time is of the essence. Time is running out, and time is apprehended more lucidly: *years suspended* by men representing police, judicial and penitentiary authority, and *years to make up for*[91]. In all cases, the very principle of the loss of the landmarks that make the sexual moment a moment of quietude and abandonment also remains a major problem. Some inmates even mention the habit of associating sexual pleasures with psychotropic drugs that are forbidden inside the

---

91. Regardless of sexual issues, where men downplay the importance of the offence they have committed, women recognize and accept the facts that landed them in prison, but declare themselves victims of a prison system that robs them of too many years. The length of incarceration, directly related to the desire for a punishment that is sufficiently dissuasive to prevent recidivism in men, is not adapted to women, whose delinquency is less professionalized. In fact, prisons are generally designed for men, based on their presumed dangerousness and current delinquency. The security measures imposed on women are undoubtedly a response to the men's desire to escape and their insubordination, but seem totally out of place when it comes to restraining a woman to go to hospital for a gynaecological examination.

Living your sexuality in prison - the missing otherness -

prison. This is the case of Jo, who has been taming his sexual arousal since he's been locked up, and for whom the deprivation of drugs, combined with the lack of sexual relations, allows him to take stock of the past few years: "With *ecstasy* and *speed*, you can hold on to desire for hours. Now when I watch porn, I don't last more than twenty minutes. There's no comparison between sex with and without drugs. [...] With the stop in prison, I realize that drugs killed me." This is also the case for Levis, for whom the novelty brought by incarceration consists in seeing sexual desire as a sentimental motor: "With the products I was taking, it helped me to get off. MDMA helps you get a hard-on, but sometimes it prevents you from ejaculating, so the sensations are less intense. Now I tell myself that the best sex drug is love."

Excitation memory

> "If, as sometimes happened, she had the features of a woman I had known in life, I was going to give myself entirely to this goal: to find her, like those who set out on a journey to see in their eyes a desired city and imagine that one can taste in reality the charm of a dream."[92]

Prisoners revive memories of past relationships in a variety of ways. It's a way of keeping alive the feeling of having existed before incarceration. Three types of reappropriation of erotic memories emerge, and the way they function enables us to apprehend the appreciation of time during long sentences. Some inmates never think about their past sex life. There are those who only think back to recent memories, sometimes limiting themselves to the last partner they loved, and sometimes still love. And there are some inmates for whom memories remain vivid without expiration. This is the case of Hippocampe: "It's still alive in me, and it's much more exciting than porn". There are also those for

---

92. PROUST (Marcel), *Du côté de chez Swann*, Paris, Gallimard, "Folio" series, 1988, p. 4.

whom memories are above all the excitements that justify their presence in prison. This is the case for Lucien, convicted of pedophilia: "When I think back, it's the memories of the girls I had fun with that come back to me. So I stop thinking about it."

In the prisoners' discourse, it is symptomatic to note that memories constitute that part of intimacy that suffers neither judgment nor judicial condemnation, inaccessible to the authority of the prison administration, and inalienable in principle. The survival of memories, as an accessory to living excitement, is akin to a resistance mechanism in the face of the symbolic death imposed by the ban on sexual relations. As Tim puts it: "I remember and it makes me travel and stop thinking that I'm in prison." Memory catches up with individuals and virtually takes them back outside. The feeling that "what you've done can still be done" is reassuring.

Erotic memories are a personal and intimate possession, the only one that prisoners know they will never be dispossessed of. Everything material in detention is subject to the surveillance power of the prison administration. Naked searches, with the body bent over to probe the contents of the rectum, attest to the omnipotence of an institution over bodies. Memories, on the other hand, are an inaccessible territory, given the current state of control techniques. The eroticism of memories represents portions of each person's life that will give new meaning to a body that wants to exult. Fantasies develop from a rewriting of the scenes experienced, according to multiple combinations that allow for an infinite variety of arousal configurations. Each person organizes his or her fantasies freely, with a view to achieving the most precise pleasure. Some relive scenes identically, while others allow themselves to reconstruct excitement scenarios, based on the circumstantial elements of the fantasy. Aside from *purely sexual* issues, memories of past relationships are also a way of rekindling amorous feelings, or at the very least, rekindling the memory of a loved and loving one. Armand claims, "Only the image of my spouse gives me a hard-on." The austerity of imprisonment gradually alters the *power to love until* these men and women are transformed into *humanoids* disembodied of humanity. Beyond libidinal arousal, the influence of memory, in the form of immaterial possession, plays a part in the survival process that each of them organizes in this universe of deprivation.

Unlike the use of pornography, identification processes are amplified by the fact that inmates are already actors in their past arousal. Tom explains: "With porn, it's more mechanical, masturbation becomes automatic." Yet the inmates who confess to reveling in their memories are also consumers of pornographic films. Awareness of the length of long sentences helps us to understand the possible exhaustion of these excitements, which by dint of being rethought too much, end up wearing out their libidinal power like a thread. By the age of 21, Augustin had already noticed that "memories are fading". These *intimate treasures* must satisfy those concerned for the duration of their incarceration. But for many, the performance of their memories deteriorates with the length of their sentences. The first break comes at the moment of incarceration, when the prisoner is set apart from society. It's an immediate and brutal break with the outside world[93]. The second break is constituted by the gradual erasure of the memory of life outside, by the increasingly definitive adaptation to life inside, which ends up being the last horizon experienced as the possibility of a life outside the walls recedes into the past.

Prisoners who are lucky enough to receive a partner in the visiting room return to their cells with renewed memories of often unconsum-

---

93. In the same vein, on the subject of the sudden rupture of sexual practices, contradicting a need thwarted by conditions beyond our control, see SEYLER (Monique), *La Prison immobile*, Paris, Desclée de Brouwer, 2001, p. 78.

mated excitement. For some, life as a couple is like this, with pleasure deferred and conjugated at a distance, as Sly describes: "In the visiting room, we have incredible desire, we leave in a state that's impossible. She masturbates when she leaves for her hotel - which is not her style - and so do I."

Prison condemns the inmate to a symbolic death from the moment of incarceration, and ratifies this elimination from society through the accumulation of years of detention, to the point of drastically reducing the prognosis for reintegration. Beyond four or five years of confinement, and assuming that a prisoner has no contact with the outside world, no visiting room or mail, long sentences are akin to a destruction of the living and the ability to exist as an individual in the social group. This is how Bruno describes his detention: "Prison excludes. If you don't have faith, education and intelligence, you're dead." In the manner of natural selection, only the strongest will survive. The maintenance of memory, among other things for libidinal purposes, is part of the work that each prisoner carries out to chronologically consider the time of incarceration, as an intermediate insularity in the course of a life.

Pornography: a substitute for the reality of the flesh

The erotic construction of prisoners has always been associated with pornographic materials. In the past, these were photos and magazines, whose prohibitive cost made them treasures of survival, dearly negotiable in detention. Today, and because it is reasonably impossible not to recognize the importance of the sexual dimension in individual wholeness, the prison administration endorses pornography as a substitute for sexuality, particularly since the authorization of televisions in cells, which took place almost simultaneously with the arrival of pornographic films on the small screen. The encrypted Canal Plus channel has, in fact, enabled the official use of pornography inside French prisons. Largely aided by the fact that the vast majority of pornography is designed to meet male expectations, redefining at the same time an assumption of omnipotent virility, of men who are always "horny", using women who are always subservient and available, pornographic encounters have become a major part of daily life in the men's prison. Of course, the harmlessness of this excitement has not been proven. We need to distinguish between inmates who will stabilize their consumption inside the house, and those who will compensate for a frustrated libido by excessive use, thereby filling not only sexual gaps, but also an idleness to which morality strives to attribute the maternity of many vices.

Criticism of this form of excitement is frequently discredited by purely moral motivations, more or less nourished by spiritual and religious inspiration, aimed at seeing pornography exclusively as a combination of perversion and regression. On the one hand, there are the *prudes* who are conservative in their conception and practice of sexuality as good fathers and fathers, and who will hurl anathemas and *cry fire* even before any danger has been identified. Assuming that pornographic situations reduce *human beings to* a bestiality long since tamed by culture, education and religion, pornography, then described as regression, is an evil to be fought, an anti-solution to questions that need to be resolved differently. On the other hand, some women adopt a feminist stance when they argue that pornography is a tool made by men, for men, while at the same time harming women, commodified to the rank of objects for the satisfaction of a virility that never ceases to be the standard value[94]. This stance is motivated by the fact that consumers of pornography would end up confusing fiction with reality. Moreover, the female supervisors we met are opposed to such practices in detention. This is the case of Angélique, who explains the danger that immoderate

---

94. In this vein, see DOMENACH (Élise), "Quels sont nos droits et nos responsabilités face à l'expression pornographique?", *Cités*, no 15, Paris, PUF, 2003, p. 99.

use of pornography can represent in a world where men accumulate a sense of frustration through the prohibition of sexual relations: "I'm against it. It turns them on, and if they're weak in the head, they can assault a matron in the morning. I heard once that a female supervisor got caught, so I'm always afraid of that kind of exception."[95]

Female inmates also have access to the pornographic material shown in the men's section of the Bapaume detention center. In the end, moral considerations aside, they expressed total indifference to these fictions, which they saw as an exclusively male tool that had nothing to do with them. Some claimed to have tried to watch on several occasions, in search of sexual arousal, only to end up preferring to do without. This is the case of Oiseau Rouge, who admits to using porn while recognizing the limits: "Sometimes I fall asleep in front of porn, but it doesn't interest me... In front of porn, I get wet, but that's it, I don't touch myself!" They declared themselves "disappointed by the lack of effect produced", unlike a majority of men who try to draw from it the revival of a virility that promises to be in disuse[96]. Marseille explains: "My husband and I write erotic literature to each other every day, but I never watch porn.

Concerns about the influence of pornography on the minds of consumers of *given and unearned arousal* become particularly acute in prisons, where pornography is no longer just a secondary form of arousal. In this case, it's a question of replacing relationships of otherness that have become impossible, with virtual identifications that deprive the individual of his or her ability to realize that the other is a thinking and

---

95. Angélique is a supervisor at the Val-de-Reuil detention center.
96. On the respective roles of men and women in the representation of pornography, see DAOUST (Valérie), *De la sexualité en démocratie. L'individu libre et ses espaces identitaires*, Paris, PUF, 2005, p. 204.

desiring being, a decision-making actor in the elements that make up the encounter, the desire, the consent and then the sexual acts themselves.

You have to imagine what it's like to have pornography in a prison. Remand prisoners mixed with convicts, first-time offenders with repeat offenders, young with old, and finally six inmates crammed together on mattresses on the floor, in a cell designed for two, sharing the same fiction without any privacy, in the religious silence of a detention entirely focused on the same TV channel. This humiliating memory remains with us, as Saul testifies: "In the prison, we shared the same cell, so we put a sheet over our heads to protect ourselves from the gaze of others when we masturbated at the same time in front of the same film. After a while, you just don't feel like jerking off anymore."

Pornographic distribution appears to be an easy, inexpensive and time-saving way of giving a false impression to men who are becoming hungrier by the day[97]. It's the institution's response to the problems posed by the deprivation of gender otherness in the context of *long-sentence* confinement. Even if technological developments have enabled the transition from printed media to television fiction, the fundamental problematic responds to identical imperatives, inherent to the very principle of prison confinement. Pornography is one of the *patches* used by the prison administration against any notion of morality or long-term objectivity. What takes precedence is the punctual, immediate effectiveness of a fact accepted as the answer to an ever-contemporary problem that needs to be dealt with on a daily basis. That's what Anne-Marie Marchetti says: "Where I perceive a dehumanizing relational void, my interlocutor (deputy director of the facility), as a pragmatic

---

97. In the same vein, the questions posed by a plant manager regarding the mission of the prison: Le Caisne (Léonore), *Prison, une ethnologue en centrale*, Paris, Odile Jacob, 2000, p. 208.

124

professional, sees only an overflow of sperm to be emptied so that on Saturday morning, the inmates are clean and relaxed, and prison life can continue its course like a long, tranquil river. De-polluted."[98]

Probably aware of the limits and drawbacks of pornography in prisons, each department reserves the right to manage the quantity and quality of fiction broadcast as it sees fit. In-house television channels show pornographic films on a daily or weekly basis, with a regular renewal of programming. This wide choice is sometimes supplemented by pornographic channels offered on satellite or cable packages. The director of a prison explains that he has recently started to monitor the quality of the DVDs[99] on offer in his establishment. While he refuses to pose as a moral censor, in a pragmatic way, he points out that we can't turn a blind eye to a pornographic market where certain trends encourage perversions that he describes as "too offbeat". He cites the case of zoophilic, pedophilic and scatophilic films. With a prison population made up of a high percentage of mentally fragile individuals, some of whom are incarcerated for sexual offenses, allowing this kind of arousal medium to circulate would be tantamount to turning a blind eye to dangerous excesses.

From the outside, the prison represents a universe in which society's prohibitions are annihilated by the walls. It is, in this sense, a place where all prohibitions become possible, a place where the superego dwindles and is transformed by the rules implicitly imposed by the

---

98. MARCHETTI (Anne-Marie), *op. cit.* p. 233.

99. The *canteen* is the prison's marketplace. It is the store where inmates can buy items and foodstuffs. Once a week, *canteen vouchers are* distributed with a list of products available for purchase. This *catalog, in the* form of a list, can range from the most ordinary foodstuffs to the most common items: food, tobacco, specific hygiene products that the prison administration would not supply, pens and papers, telephone cards, magazines and newspapers, pornographic DVDs. Certain products are prohibited, such as alcohol, lighters, etc.

Living your sexuality in prison - the missing otherness -

monosexual universe. Guilt, far from disappearing, becomes lighter, or takes on a face full of justifications linked to the contingencies of confinement. The absence of the inquisitive gaze of family and friends, to whom inmates cannot displease, plunges consciences into a system where values are transformed, to conform only to the prescriptions of a single-gender community. For other inmates, the desire not to *get dirty*, not to become something they weren't before entering prison, acts as a censor of individual behavior. Augustin explains: "I had my TV removed because of the porn. I wanted to smash the TV because, in fact, people in pornos are like animals." Charles corroborates: "Pornography is destructive, it affects the psyche of people who already have problems. I don't think it gives a true image of man, the overpowering man and the whore woman!" Just as some inmates invest money and physical effort to keep their bodies in shape during detention, others are concerned with maintaining their self-image as intact as possible for the duration of their incarceration. This requires an inordinate amount of patience, extraordinary willpower and unfailing optimism, in order to maintain a projection of oneself onto a horizon that may be decades away. It's also the characterization of a dignity that inmates refuse to concede to the prison institution, out of consideration for themselves with a view to release, but also out of survival resistance to an authoritarian regime they challenge. Charles explains: "In prison, there are two ways of surviving: either enter the system, with the risk of losing who you are, or do only what you are forced to do. I corresponded with Jorge Semprun, who also survived with this same approach to the system, refusing all logic. He even refused to let bars be bars."[100]

As with the consumption of psychotropic drugs offered by the medical-psychiatric service, the aim for long-sentence prisoners is often to

---

100. Charles, 54, sentenced to life imprisonment for voluntary manslaughter, is being held in Val-de-Reuil.

avoid adding a liberticidal dependency to the deprivation of freedom imposed by incarceration. For some, *remaining free within the walls of confinement is* the most elaborate form of resistance they can muster to preserve a few bulwarks of dignity in the midst of a humiliating institution. It's not so much an unconditional submission to the deprivation of sexual relations, as a refusal to submit to the only palliative offered by the prison administration, a palliative that would replace the bromide of the past. Like the superego, to which Freud attributes the virtue of "developing autonomy"[101], independence from prison constraints is an achievement of freedom, signifying that the prisoner refuses to allow himself to be so objectified by an alienating system.

The pornographic consumption observed among certain fellow inmates - and the obsession that goes with it - represents one of the many excesses that imprisonment encourages, and is a reminder of the survival mechanisms that everyone develops to counter what Freud described as anguish "in reaction to the loss of object"[102]. Mr. T., a long-time inmate of a detention center housing a large majority of sex offenders, has this to say about pornographic films: "People convicted of rape have complained to the shrinks, telling them that porn films arouse them too much, that they can't correct themselves. So the shrinks got two out of four channels removed. In fact, some people are so obsessed with porn that they set the alarm in the middle of the night to make sure they don't miss the broadcast."

For some inmates in couples, the use of pornography is a form of infidelity. Seeing one's partner in the visiting room at weekends, only to become aroused by an unknown woman whose scripted behavior has no resemblance to reality, ends up disrupting the feeling of being

---

101. FREUD (Sigmund), "Des types libidinaux", in *Œuvres complètes*, Paris, PUF, 1995, p. 5.
102. FREUD (Sigmund), *Inhibition, Symptom and Anguish*, Paris, PUF, 1993, p. 81.

in a couple. Doudou, a prisoner in Val-de-Reuil, who has been in a relationship for four years with a woman he met through a classified ad, explains: "I have few ways of showing my faithfulness to my girlfriend. So not looking at other women on TV is the least I can do, knowing that outside she has solicitations she doesn't respond to."

In the end, the excitement produced by pornography in detention has more to do with satisfying and encouraging voyeuristic impulses, than with the illusory substitution of a carnal relationship. Some claim to be obsessed by exponential pornographic consumption, going so far as to accumulate an impressive DVD library. Others make do with Canal Plus's monthly porno, which is recognized as unedited and of better quality. The *other films* all look the same, according to Marcus, himself a former porn actor, "and in the end, the characters never get married!" The broadcasting times don't seem to suit inmates who have a profes-sional life in detention, which seems to attest to the importance of a regulating activity during the sentence. This is the case for Jo: "I watch porn once a month, but only at weekends. During the week I don't have time, I work and have to get up early."

To sum up, pornography in prison is not without its share of para-doxes. The majority of inmates are shocked by the lack of credibility of an institution which, on the one hand, prohibits sexual relations between couples, and, on the other hand, feeds arousal through the daily distribution[103] of pornography, particularly for the benefit of a population of sex offenders.

---

103. Many detention centers have in-house television channels. Sometimes run by a team of inmates, these in-house channels can also broadcast pornographic films, in competi-tion with cable channels and Canal Plus. Finally, even if broadcasting times don't allow everyone to watch TV at all hours, the offer is daily.

The need for pleasure and the need for pain

In this paradoxical situation of sexual deprivation combined with imprisonment, where no moral concept[104] justifies abstinence from sexual pleasure, the promotion of masturbation *via* pornography exacerbates practices in which all those involved in prison life are *de facto accomplices*. Doctors and nurses are frequently called in to treat the damage caused by over-intense masturbation, sometimes akin to forms of self-mutilation, which, beyond being motivated by demands or expressions of despair, also contain an assumed libidinal dimension. This is the case for Franck, for example, when he says: "I use dildos, or objects covered with a sock and then a condom (a bottle of household cleaner). I try not to overdo it, because I can get too big, and that leads to pain, which isn't healthy for me. The problem with self-destruction is that you tell yourself you're worthless, that you're going to destroy yourself. It's a masochistic pleasure, different from anal sex."

Psychologist Simone Buffard notes a direct correlation between wrist self-mutilation and the guilt generated by feelings of adolescent regression, for these men who are condemned to the deprivation of adult sexuality[105]. Daniel Gonin analyzes self-mutilation as an ultimate means of satisfying impulsive needs, which the inmates experience as a combination of frustration and despair[106]: "This practice [penetrating a bloody hole in the plaster of the wall] appeared to us in its obstinacy as a voluntary mutilation, a kind of amputation of enjoyment, a suicidal equivalent without equal."[107]

---

104. RUBIN (Gayle S.), *op. cit.* p. 84.
105. BUFFARD (Simone), *Le Froid pénitentiaire. L'impossible réforme des prisons*, Paris, Le Seuil, coll. "Esprit", 1973, p. 44.
106. On frustration tolerance, see PICHOT (Pierre) and DANJON (Suzanne), *Le Test de frustration de Rosenzweig*, Paris, Éditions du Centre de psychologie appliquée, 1966, p. 5.
107. GONIN (Daniel), *op. cit.* p. 160.

So, far from being a morally reprehensible practice, the substitution of masturbation for sexual relations appears to be a perverse phenomenon, not from a psychological point of view, but for the long-term consequences that the missing otherness imprints on the progressive inability to be another's self. Behind the frenzy of practices that remind us of the possibility of a sexuality kept alive, lie dependencies and mutilations of the body, which underline that in sexual matters too, the measure in compensating for lack proves a perilous exercise without the landmarks of otherness. Orgasmic pleasure and ejaculation do not simply replace coitus. The function of masturbation concentrates the shortcomings of sexuality in its broadest sense. Encounter, seduction, tenderness and genital pleasure all have to find expression in the unique opportunity of solitary sexual practice.

THIRD PART

TENTATIONS AND DANGERS
OF CARCERAL HOMOSEXUALITY
- Otherness forbidden -

"The teachers who, for centuries, taught children how intolerable homosexuality was and who purged literature textbooks, falsified history in order to exclude this type of sexuality, have caused more havoc than the teacher who talks about homosexuality and can do no other harm than explain a given reality, a lived experience."[108]

In a monosexual world, when it comes to sexual relations, the choice of partner can only be made between individuals of the same sex. That's why the myth of the *soapbox picked up in the shower is so* enduring. Yet homophobia is actually more present than homosexuality in the institutions of penal repression. Far from the rampant fantasy of a society which, through ignorance of prison reality, allows the rumor to persist that all inmates end up being homosexual, homophobia is skilfully nurtured in prisons.

Does imprisonment cause the majority of inmates to slide from an impossible heterosexuality to a homosexuality of circumstance or substitution? This is an idea that is as widespread as it is falsely established, claiming that all prisoners become homosexual during the course of their imprisonment. It's also a further argument for maintaining vigo-

---

108. FOUCAULT (Michel), *Dits et écrits*, Paris, Gallimard, 1994.

rous homophobia behind bars. Men who are locked up take a dim view of the idea that they have slipped, on the inside, into practices they would have disapproved of on the outside. Women, on the other hand, are relatively free to engage in practices that do not call their reputation into question. In prison, homophobia takes on the specific characteristics of a predominantly masculine gender posture.

So, whatever the sexual practices carried out in makeshift alcoves, verbalizing the unspeakable would be tantamount to acknowledging what one cannot assume. So it's customary to express disdain and even hatred of homosexuals, to ensure that you officially keep a safe distance from the *kind of men you* refuse to become, and in whose company it's always better not to be seen. In the prison economy, sharing a cell, or even the friendship of a recognized homosexual, is akin to admitting one's masculinity is in danger.

Since it has become less moral[109], homophobia expresses the persistence of a sometimes visceral fear in group relations. It's not so much the fear of homosexuals as what they are, but rather the danger they represent for the image they give of virility. In the prison world, homosexuals are often equated with rapists and pedophiles. They belong to this hierarchical category of ostracized beings. However, the latitude allowed for the expression of homosexuality differs from one prison to another, depending on the configuration of the premises, the prison governor and the prerogatives acquired by inmates as a result of an ongoing power struggle with the prison administration. In practice, male homosexuality is very frequently linked to violence, acts of possession and domination, a whole arsenal satisfying relationships of force and interest, mostly devoid of seduction and affect. The question of the

---

109. In this sense, and with a scientific argument, see RUBIN (Gayle S.), *op. cit.* p. 85.

informed consent of sexual partners remains the prison administration's main problem. And if a hierarchy of acceptability is established for homosexual behavior, it's only to emphasize that a man remains a man when he penetrates.

Chapter 1
Homophobia in detention

"In the beginning, there's the insult. The one that every gay man can hear at some point in his life, and which is the sign of his psychological and social vulnerability."[110]

The psychological mechanism of fear comes into play as a means of defense against presumed or actual aggression. Phobias are sometimes considered to be uncontrollable manifestations, often obeying no rationality other than Annie Birraux's definition of the *memory of fear*[111]. On the contrary, homophobia in prison rationally responds to an imperative of resistance to the sexual behavior that the deprivation of heterosexuality in *long sentences inevitably* provokes. This is Michel Bozon's definition of the licit and illicit, which makes some people censors of the illicit acts of others[112]. In subtle doses, the desire for punishment is expressed through bullying, insults and humiliations that stigmatize the reproached difference. In lethal doses, phobias underpin the destruction of the object of fear. The words collected during the interviews reveal a violence, verbalized on the one hand

---

110. ERIBON (Didier), *Réflexions sur la question gay*, Paris, Fayard, 1999, p. 29.
111. BIRRAUX (Annie), *Éloge de la phobie*, Paris, PUF, 1994, p. 14.
112. BOZON (Michel), *Sociologie de la sexualité*, Paris, Armand Colin, 2005, p. 14.

and acted out on the other, through physical as well as moral aggression: "These people are atrocious - insults are all they deserve - homos risk a beating at any moment." In both cases, homophobia is a denial, whether asserted or not, that comes to soothe a fear that ravages, according to argued developments whose origins lie in history, morality, social representations of gender, scientific interpretation and spiritual presuppositions.

The power of homophobia through the law of numbers

In prison institutions, as in the outside world, the norm is defended above all by the *law of numbers*, which alone enables the arguments developed to define heterosexuality as the inescapable standard of the economies of desire[113] to survive, so as to isolate *order from chaos*[114]. This creates a balance of power between the defenders of the norm and those who have supposedly gone astray, which a restrictive arsenal will take on the task of reframing. Homosexuals are in the minority, and their social recognition, in the economy of power relations in detention, is subject to physical and verbal violence, in relations of domination and negation. Wesley, a prisoner at Œrmingen, explains: "Some of them can get stabbed. They're never at peace here. Max admits that, "on the outside, gays are more diluted". As *coming out* is accompanied by the risk of violence, the authority of homophobia, held by the beneficiaries of the *law of numbers*, subjects homosexuals to silence, and to *self-denial* through the denial of their own desires.

---

113. On the presumed evolution of the concept of norm with regard to sexual orientation: "[...] it is perhaps not completely absurd to think that one day, heterosexuality, having become detached from the biological needs of reproduction, will require certain explanations", DAOUST (Valérie), *De la sexualité en démocratie. L'individu libre et ses espaces identitaires*, Paris, PUF, 2005, p. 175.
114. RUBIN (Gayle S.), *op. cit.* p. 89.

In the Caen detention center, the stakes are very different. With a sex offender population approaching 80%, the law of numbers doesn't favor the camp of kingpins and other robbers, but rather the usually reviled *sexual minorities.* Pointers and homosexuals, strengthened by their numerical representation, subvert the norm and invalidate the coercive power of heterosexual supremacy. Hervé, a prisoner in Caen, says: "When the kids have fun calling us fags, we calm them down and put them in their place." So when a detention center director explains that allowing sexual relations between inmates would entail too many risks of aggression and submission, this argument falls flat at the Caen center. That's why relations between fellow inmates are tacitly authorized, to the point of being made possible by a mechanism of curtains and hooks, to protect the modesty of guards and inmates, during the *daytime open regime.* This pragmatic arrangement meets the requirements of *modesty* and the *sanctioning of obscenity* imposed by the Code of Criminal Procedure[115]. The economy of power, when it is not nourished by the weapons of authority consisting in the threat of destruction by force, when it is not globalized in perfect totalitarianism, relies on the economy of numbers, mathematically quantified under the term *majority.* This situation is reminiscent of the will to power described by Nietzsche[116], when he recognizes the capacity of the *weak* to become dominant, to the point of oppressing the strong who are in the minority. This is the balance of power that emerges at the Caen detention center, where the power of the norm and the coercion of the

115. Once a day, at a set time, supervisors visit the cells to probe the bars. A supervisor opens the door of each cell, to which a fellow inmate delivers the canteen. Apart from these visits, and unless you are under special surveillance or have been summoned to see a chief, the open regime allows you to receive a partner discreetly in your individual cell.

116. NIETZSCHE (Friedrich), *Beyond Good and Evil,* Paris, Aubier, 1978. See also "Posthumous Fragments", vol. XII, notebook WI 8, 1886-1887, in *Œuvres philosophiques complètes,* Paris, Gallimard, 1967-1997.

defenders of male heterosexuality are defused by the group of *degraded* and *weak,* made up of pointers and homosexuals.

The specifics of homophobia in women's prisons

"How can you punish something that doesn't exist?" a question attributed to Queen Victoria on the issue of impunity for sexual relations between women.

There are major differences between men's and women's experiences of homosexuality, and these lead to significant variations in homophobic expression. The main difference lies in the fact that homosexuality does not seem to be a matter of identity for women, and is not limited to a carnal association aimed at procuring an orgasm. It's often more an opportunity for tenderness, caresses and cuddles, naturally seized as a substitute for solitude in a monosexual universe. This sexual orientation, often accompanied by emotional involvement, does not call into question the female gender identity. Women don't lose the attributes that society grants them when they get romantically or carnally involved with another woman. All they do is fall into a non-conformist attitude with regard to a heterosexual norm, which they flout with a disorder that has no consequences for the image of women. Marie-Françoise, an inmate at Bapaume, sums up the main reticence when the desire or need for a carnal relationship arises: "I gave it up out of loyalty to my husband, but it would have been possible." In the end, women appear freer in their ability to *exist differently,* insofar as they have neither the ambition nor the need to defend an illusion of power whose absence would disqualify them. In fact, there are many official couples in women's detention centers, and their existence as much as their serenity is not due to the tolerance of the law of numbers, but rather to an acquired and genera-lized liberality. Provided women's attitudes towards each other are not too demonstrative, female couples can ask to be *doubled up,* i.e. to live

Tentations and dangers of carceral homosexuality - otherness forbidden -

together in the same cell. In some prisons, the prison administration makes every effort to accommodate requests for pairing up, without ever raising the question of couples and sexuality. Officially, therefore, these *doublets do* not constitute proof of a homosexual couple.

This contrasting tolerance in relation to the detention of men, does not exclude insults, bullying and other expressions of disagreement, perceived as attenuated, non-stigmatizing homophobia. Conflicting relationships have no identity connotations, and carry little more weight than criticism of any physical detail. In female detention, homosexual relationships are trivialized as anecdotes with no major consequences, so homophobia is limited to highlighting one difference rather than another. With detachment and hindsight, Béatrice, an inmate at Bapaume, recalls an experience that was as uninhibited as it was guilt-free: "I tried it with a woman, but it didn't work, it was the first time, and I don't want to go back there. Bickering" does not rule out sudden friendly reversals. Myriam, an inmate at Bapaume, limits her opinion on the homosexual question to: "It doesn't bother me, there's nothing wrong with doing yourself good! Where there's pleasure, there's no embarrassment." On the other hand, the constant infidelities of *lovers*, the ensuing fits of jealousy and possessive relationships, make homosexuality seem like an untamed deviance, with no connection whatsoever with the stakes of a heterosexual relationship. Myriam, an inmate at Bapaume, notes: "They insult each other and it makes them sick. Executioners know what to do with their victims!"

The gradations of homophobia obey an assessment of the consequences, sometimes objective, sometimes subjective. Of course, daily insults and bullying in women's prisons are less damaging than rapes or other manifestations of hatred that can even lead to death in men's prisons. However, the reclassification of homophobia based on the minimization of its consequences should not lead us to overlook the stigmatization

140

on which it is based, at the risk of scorning the very existence of the principle of discrimination, as real as it is insidious. For a long time, authors dealing with the carnal rapprochement between women only defined a pseudo-homosexuality[117], while men were irreversibly stigmatized as *homosexuals.* This difference still seems to prevail in women's relationships in prison, and attests to a hierarchy in sexual behavior.

The specifics of homophobia in men's prisons

In prison, male homophobia is more prevalent than female homophobia, because the stakes of what men do or don't do are paramount in a vision of society in which men must be dominant and women subordinate. For men, violence against homosexuals is powerful and authoritarian. It becomes normative through the coercion it imposes, the fear it generates, and the damage it causes[118]. Homophobia is an instrument of power, since it protects the symbolic value of masculine power, defended by a gender community whose members fear that the devaluation of the collective will result in the devaluation of the individual. The fear of degradation is an admission of individual weakness, and the signature of the postulate that the power identified in men can only be sustained by the solidarity of all. Implicitly, it's a recognition that the power vested in masculinity is little more than the sum of individual powers.

It's not so much the concept of pleasure and happiness in conjugating one's being with someone of the same sex as oneself that is being

---

117. In his book *Psychopathia sexualis*, R. von Krafft-Ebing notes that "all the information that can be gleaned from the specialized literature clearly demonstrates that in women, it is rarely a question of authentic homosexuality, but rather of pseudo-homosexuality". See also: BUTLER (Judith) and RUBIN (Gayle S.), *Marché au sexe*, Paris, Epel, 2001, p. 38.
118. FALCONNET (Georges) and LEFAUCHEUR (Nadine), *La Fabrication des mâles*, Paris, Le Seuil, 1975, p. 90.

challenged in prison today. Similarly, it's not the image of the sexual relationship, in terms of carnal practice, that's frightening. The stumbling block to homophobia in prison lies more in the representation that each person makes of it, and from which it is difficult to escape in a closed, monosexual environment. It's the symbolism of the degradation of men's image that contradicts cultural conceptions of masculinity. All the circumstances behind homosexual behavior reveal the degradation of masculine power. The individual stakes lie in maintaining a collective reputation as much as in preserving a self-image reflected in the gaze of others likely to recognize and sanction homosexual inclinations. Tom, a prisoner at Œrmingen, says he's open to socializing with homosexuals, yet he admits: "When you're in a cell with a gay or bi person, the neighbors and the way others look at you mean you have to change cells to avoid tarnishing your straight reputation." In fact, when questioned individually, many people today feel: "Everyone does as they please", "it's not our place to judge", "I know some people personally, and it doesn't bother me". But repositioned in a monosexual universe, these same inmates take on a mission of their own, that of being the preservers of true virility in the men's prison.

The cultural argument of the maison-des-hommes

Since the advent of "modern industrial societies", Michel Foucault has emphasized "the manifest explosion of heretical sexualities, [...] the proliferation of specific pleasures and the multiplication of disparate sexualities"[119]. With the gradual erosion of the influence of religious ideologies[120], it was a matter of preserving the reputation of a sex, embo-

---

119. FOUCAULT (Michel), *Histoire de la sexualité I. La volonté de savoir*, Paris, Gallimard, 1976, p. 67.
120. When it comes to homosexuality, it's not so much the precepts of the Catholic Church that have evolved, as the legitimacy accorded by believers to moral judgments emanating from the Vatican. See BORRILLO (Daniel), *L'Homophobie*, Paris, PUF, coll. "Que sais-je?", 2000, p. 49.

died by a *gender*, whose capacity for power and domination remained a standard value. The judgment of homosexuality in prison feeds on the evolution of society on the outside, with a chronological lag and an additional brake[121]. Above all, it's a question of defending the men's prison as a *conservatory of masculinity*, which allows neither compromise nor submission. Henri, an inmate at Val-de-Reuil, notes: "Violence against gays is to protect the world of men. I know one here, but he's in a closed environment, so we forget about him because we don't see him." Prison imposes the need to be a man among men: virility is an obligatory value, connived at by men reacting to a homosociality whose presumed consequences they are trying to combat. Fabrice confides: "In prison, I have to make sure I'm more virile than I am outside." Manliness serves as a virtue when homosexuality, too often associated with pedophilia, represents the *axis of evil*. Male virtue does not exclude vindictiveness and violence carried out in defiance of the law, insofar as the defense of masculinity is erected, individually and collectively, as a non-negotiable value to be protected whatever the cost. The phallus is a symbol of power, and any posture of submission is predatory of the very essence of the *male attitude*. Power and domination are defended by the male collectivity as two ontological characteristics of their gender. All sexual practices, as well as relational behaviors, which might jeopardize this culturally acquired reputation in a male-dominated society, are repressed out of *duty*.

Prison, through the authority it exerts over men, and the autonomy it removes from those it confines, distorts the face of masculinity. These phenomena are added to the arguments that, outside, motivate homophobia, defined as "discrimination against people who display,

---

121. In the same vein, and on the evolution of moral issues relating to sexuality, see Lo-CHAK (Danièle), "La liberté sexuelle, une liberté (pas) comme les autres?", *in* BORRILLO (Daniel) and LOCHAK (Danièle), (eds.), *La Liberté sexuelle*, Paris, PUF, 2005, p. 31.

or to whom is attributed, certain qualities (or defects) attributed to the other gender"[122]. Male prisoners have this additional reason to set up homophobia as a system for protecting the attributes of one gender. Submissiveness, as opposed to power, is sanctioned by the guardians of masculinity. The sanctions inflicted begin with the stigmatization of individuals with insults that serve as identification. At a second level of prejudice, homophobia takes the form of violence and domination. In both cases, it signifies the absolute prohibition of men from emancipating themselves from the cultural definition of what society expects of them. This need for normalization is not unrelated to the fact that prison clientele are mainly from the working classes[123], more inclined, according to Richard Hoggart, to the persistence of norms[124].

Resistance to the permissiveness of the outside world

Since its decriminalization in 1982[125], homosexuality has acquired an inescapable status in the public space of mainstream society. The visibility of homosexuality appears almost systematically in written or filmed fiction. Yesterday's scandal is fading behind today's trivialization. Even if some inmates are particularly vehement about these moral excesses that "herald the end of civilization": "I don't understand, I'm against it, it's inhuman what they're doing, it's disgusting. They [homosexuals]

---

122. WELZER-LANG (Daniel), *in* BORRILLO (Daniel), *L'Homophobie*, op. cit. p. 17
123. According to the INSEE survey published in 2000, one prisoner in seven has never held a job, and one in two is or has been a blue-collar worker, compared with one in three in the general population. Conversely, senior executives are under-represented in prison: they account for 3.3% of the prison population.
124. HOGGART (Richard), *The Culture of the Poor*, Paris, Éditions de Minuit, 1970
125. Under the presidency of François Mitterrand, and in the government of Pierre Mauroy, Robert Badinter submitted to the Assembly the decriminalization of homosexuality, which was achieved in France on July 27, 1982, with the repeal of article 332-1 of the Penal Code. Nine years later, in 1991, the World Health Organization (WHO) removed homosexuality from the list of mental illnesses.

should all be put in prison! Even the women!"[126] We need to distinguish between moral homophobia, which forces us to punish, and protective homophobia, which is skilfully maintained to preserve the status of men in a monosexual prison system.

The deep-rooted motivations behind the hatred of homosexuals in detention stem from a skilful cocktail of self-perception and exposure to others. The arguments put forward are fuelled by a combination of hatred and fear, identical to that which prevailed on the outside, when the PACS was adopted[127], motivating discrimination expressed under "faggots to the stake" signs, which would probably never have gone unpunished had it been a question of skin color or religious affiliation. In some of the speeches we heard, gay marriages and the adoption of children by homosexual couples were seen as *aberrations*, *deviances* and a *degeneration of* human behavior. Doudou, incarcerated in Val-de-Reuil, explains his vision of society in the face of the new prerogatives claimed or acquired by homosexuals in the outside world: "Gay marriages and adoption by gay couples, it's ugly and vile! It's an incitement to degeneration. Incarceration has aggravated my rejection of fags."

Beyond the homophobia instrumentalized for the male condition, these opinions attest to the involvement of prisoners in a society from which they are nonetheless temporarily extracted. Behind some of the speeches is the fear that, through the acceptance of new mores, an established heterosexual order will be supplanted by a new homosexual order. With the underlying fear of not finding their place in society, as

---

126. "Prisoner Prof", 27, incarcerated in OErmingen for drug trafficking. Practicing Muslim.

127. The PACS or Civil Solidarity Pact, conceived as a marriage with reduced effects, enables two people of the same sex to obtain certain prerogatives of spouses (law 99-944 of November 15, 1999).

heterosexuals, of not recognizing, in the hour of liberation, this outside society that would have changed to their disadvantage. As Daniel Borrilllo writes[128], homophobia is consciously used as a bulwark against the imagined disappearance of reproductive heterosexuality, in favor of sterile homosexuality.

The risks posed by homosexual practices in detention, whether they concern physical or mental integrity, are all dissuasive ideas, developed on the basis of inflicted or potential suffering, according to the dissuasive model of the punitive nature of prison. The risk of judicial sanction to dissuade disobedience to the law outside echoes the risk of violence to dissuade disobedience to the heterosexual norm inside. The *homosexual evil*, in semantic and conceptual opposition to the *homosexual male*, is defined as a disease, provoking an assimilation with the *pedophile evil*. The fear sometimes expressed in interviews is that of a numerical battle between heterosexuality and homosexuality, in which victory for homosexuals would force heterosexuals to annex themselves to practices they disapprove of. The same Doudou worries about a proliferation of homosexuality, which only homophobic behavior could regulate: "I fear a total collapse of love and sentimental values, afraid that in the end straight people will be singled out. It's a form of mental illness. For women, I'm more tolerant."

Homophobia or the resistance of the weakened

While underlining the precariousness of men's symbolic power, prison homophobia reconstitutes its myth. Perceived as a consequence of confinement, homosexuality in prison is unbearable insofar as it embodies submission to the institution. It's not so much that the prison administration generates or sustains hatred of homosexuals, even if some warders sometimes position themselves as guardians of

---

128. BORRILLO (Daniel), *op. cit.* p. 6.

the phallus. Above all, by making heterosexual coitus impossible, prisons castrate the phallus by organizing a regression to *non-adult status*. Submission to the prison regime, the constraints of daily obedience to the authority of the prison administration, sometimes embodied by men, sometimes by women, are all submissions that erode day after day the ability to feel powerful. This precariousness of masculinity is perceived as a danger that is accentuated by the presence and association of homosexuals. They represent the embodiment of a lost reality, of a failure that prison is a daily reminder of. Marwik, an inmate at Saint-Mihiel, explains his own vigilance in the face of behavior he'd rather not adopt: "I know it's possible for me, but I hold back. It's weakness that makes us accept. I've surprised myself by thinking I was going off the rails. Everyone runs that risk when their sex life breaks down. I was able to dominate myself because I'm against it. I imagined myself in the role of a man... Today, I bump into them, so I say hello, but no more."

Prison homophobia does not borrow all the factors of homophobia on the outside. Some of its motivations have to do with the very principle of confinement and the humiliations that detention generates. The lost phallus is the *extinguished torch* carried by these men, degraded once by the expression of their condemnation, twice by the relegation to which they are subjected, three times by the power they lose over women, four times by submission to prison authority. A fifth humiliation would be one too many: we must fight this homosexuality, which is casting a shadow over an already seriously tarnished reputation. So, when the degradation of masculinity becomes the collective cause of keeping males in a heterosexual orientation, the resistance consists in reproducing the ostracism of Greek cities: "When two tough guys are caught in the showers, they ask for isolation and then for their transfer; nobody talks to them anymore. It's a neo-fascist society here, with all kinds of racism superimposed on each other: against pointers, gays, this or that ethnic group...".[129] The prison institution is a producer of homophobia, not so much as an objective, but as a consequence of the very principles that govern its existence. Homophobia appears to be the side-effect of a system which, because it undermines a sense of virility, generates individual and collective conflicts, both mental and physical, whose resolution can only be envisaged through violence and domination.

Domination hidden behind tolerance

Prisoners' pathologizing discourse on homosexuality has also authorized a *discourse of choice*, a *choice to be and* not a *choice to live what one is*. Prison homophobia recognizes *theoretical freedom of choice*, but prevents *freedom of practice*. In prison, homosexuality is as frightening as it is incomprehensible, as if it were an option fundamentally interchangeable with heterosexuality through the exercise of free will. This idea, which is widespread beyond prison walls, means that tolerance towards homosexuals is seen as a favor, not a principle. Thus, in prison, homosexuals are indebted to heterosexuals for the altruism the latter demonstrate when they allow the possible choice of a marginal sexual orientation to develop.

Paradoxically, some inmates explained that homophobia was less intense in detention than in society outside. According to them, this point of view is justified by the learning of tolerance, mostly defined as an inescapable result of confinement, which gradually feeds an apprenticeship in homosociality. This is the case of Hervé, a prisoner convicted of homophobic violence, who was led to modify his point of view following an encounter with a fellow inmate: "Then, in the third year of detention, a boy eight years younger than me shared my cell. He was gay, and he told me that homosexuality was good. He taught

---

129. MARCHETTI (Anne-Marie), *op. cit.* p. 249.

me about caresses and gentleness. He helped me discover that it could be done with a lot of tolerance and, combined with the work with the shrink, I ended up accepting my homosexuality."

Prison forces a social mix. How, over the years, can you tirelessly reproach the same people for the same things? What is the value of forced tolerance? Eventually, the human differences that prison imposes become too much to bear. In some cases, unreasoned tolerance, acquired through resignation, leads to a greater acceptance of other people's homosexuality than outside. Wolf, who we met outside the prison walls, explains the tolerance he has acquired towards homosexuality: "Imagine a small space with several people, you inevitably become more tolerant. To survive, you have to accept. I've become more tolerant than before, more patient too, but that's thanks to prison. Outside, you can move to another town if you don't like someone. In prison, you have to put up with it, so you get used to it."

Behind this tolerance lies homophobia. Bruno, an inmate at Val-de-Reuil, explains the dual behavior he combines to avoid jeopardizing a tolerance that remains precarious: "I talk about it with some people, more and more even. But with everyone else, I'm straight." When it suddenly becomes urgent to reaffirm one's own heterosexuality within the group, tolerance cannot be analyzed as a moral posture. It's more the result of a pragmatic attitude linked to the forced mixing of differences in a restricted space. The serenity of homosexuals in detention is therefore relative. It depends on the moods and stakes of those who authorize it. In any case, at best, homosexuals remain subject to the power of the *law of numbers*, the defenders of the heterosexual male world, who choose despotically and arbitrarily to tolerate or insult, defend or violate. This situation thrives on the perpetual uncertainty of seeing complicity turn into denunciation, exchange into violence, and friendship into ostracism. Here again, sexuality is a unifying factor in relationships of power and domination. Prison tolerance is part of the power that inmates grant themselves to dominate their fellow inmates. It acts as a *power of grace* that remains the prerogative of those who hold the power to normalize.

An antidote to individual homosexual desires

When heterosexuality becomes shaky, the personal ban on homosexual practices is jeopardized by the lightness with which other inmates *succumb to* them. This is an illustration of a *commonplace*, both globalizing and undeniable, summarizing homophobia as manifestations of violence emanating from individuals who do not accept their own share of homosexuality. As outside, prison homophobia acts as a normalizing regulation of the presumed expansion of homosexuality. Doudou admits: "You need homophobes to prevent homosexuality from spreading too far, it's a plague." Like *mantras* repeated tirelessly, homophobic speeches, as much as the standardized behavior of homophobia in prison, act as a commitment not to succumb to homosexuality, to the point of reinforcing a collectively defined and protected prohibition. Behind the protection of representations of the male group also lies the protection of individual narcissistic images. Homophobic obsession serves to maintain an individual carapace in the face of desires forbidden in the house of men.

Ryan recalls the radical nature of his relationship with homosexuals: "If I'd been queer, I'd have said fuck everyone, but since I'm not, they all disgust me." His disgust with homosexuals nonetheless authorized him to masturbate with several people, "but with each one having his own sex!", to have relationships mixing several boys and girls, "but without having homosexual relations", and to have fellatio performed by men outside prison: "It sucked, it disgusted me [...] but I did it again with someone else another time." His discourse never ceased to address homosexuality in the form of a curiosity acted out in his past sexual behavior, and verbalized in questions. At the same time, he was radical

in his views on homosexuality, going so far as to assert that "a raped man
is always a consenting man". In his eyes, the submissiveness of some
men is a state of affairs that justifies their classification as *sub-human*,
assimilable to women, and therefore penetrable at will.

Publicly denigrating homosexuality constitutes a public commitment
to differentiate oneself from those one criticizes. Homophobia expressed
in this way acts as a *profession of faith* that formalizes radical heterosexuality, as a challenge to all, which pride will take up when libido comes
to sow doubt. Homophobia thus weaves a close link between a promise
kept by the word of the male, and homosexual attractions towards
which one cannot slip. Homophobia in detention is skilfully nurtured
to lend credibility to a heterosexuality which, although displayed as
exclusive, is sometimes seriously eroded over the years. Léon, an inmate
at Val-de-Reuil, admits: "Being homophobic means not accepting your
homosexuality. In the end, homophobia in prison reassures only those
who practice it. No one seems to be fooled by the outrageous hatred and
discrimination directed at homosexuals. As in the outside world, any
excessively verbose speech is quickly suspected of being an admission of
unacknowledged homosexuality. Armand, an inmate at Val-de-Reuil,
explains: "Homophobia is used to convince us that we're tough and
macho. And the more homophobic they seem, the more queer they are,
like the natural average of people on the outside!" And the only people
who don't realize the clarity of these unconscious admissions are often
those whose need to be homophobic obscures any self-criticism.

The normative confinement of confinement

In contrast to the diluting power of urban masses, the prison represents
a social group reduced in number, restricted in space and limited in
access. Reactions are exacerbated, and confinement produces a concentration of issues that has no equal in society outside. Homophobia is
intensified by this lack of escape, making opposition more violent.

Conflicts can't be defused by fleeing, since there's no such thing as *elsewhere*. Alfred, a prisoner at Œrmingen, points out that "you can't escape homophobia like you can outside, where there's always a place where gays are accepted". Like all institutions based on the principle of confinement, prisons confine individuals to the point of pressurizing them in an airtight, valve-less system. Mutinies, escapes and all forms of rebellion come to mind, representing an overflow of *indigestible excesses* suffered by a population that is exhausted trying to contain itself. Faced with this contingency, the best defense for homosexuals is discretion, "non-existence" at the heart of detention. Following the rule of "the less you know, the less you say", homosexuals in prison gain a pseudo-serenity through self-effacement. This denial of *who they are is a* testament to the effectiveness of homophobia, one of whose aims is precisely to eradicate those *defects* that would mar the reputation of virility. Because they have no place in the prison public space, they keep a low profile, to the extent that some of those we met confessed to hiding their homosexuality for many years in detention. Other inmates spoke of the difficulty of identifying homosexuals, who "don't have it written on them who they are". Everyone is aware that a revelation can prove fatal in a world from which there is no escape.

It's the authenticity of heterosexuality, as a natural reproductive system, that reassures us. Authenticity is equated with naturalness, understood as a law that escapes human influence. This is where inmates place the truth, in an entity external to man, translated into multiple spiritualities capable of moralizing behavior. Their worldview is binary. There's the heterosexual norm on one side, and perversions on the other. This conception is supported by the reference that Marwik, a prisoner in Val-de-Reuil, expresses: "God created woman with Adam's rib."[130]

---

130. "Book of Genesis", chapter II, verses 21-25, The Jerusalem Bible, *op. cit.*, p. 19.

Homosexuality recalls the debate on order and disorder as an allegory of the origin of chaos in the human species. In prison, it provokes disorder through the aggression it arouses, and through the assimilation of homosexuality with sexual offenses. As Bruno, an inmate at Val-de-Reuil, puts it: "I'm angry with the fascists, who want to break pointers and faggots."

When it comes to homophobia, the penitentiary institution reminds us that reduced space is normative, while extended space is prescriptive. The confinement of incarceration normalizes violent repression against individuals, whose attitude degrades phallic power, with regard to a heterosexual norm claimed to be timeless and universal. Because the prison world is closed, because the deprivation of sexual relations is perceived as a lack for which no satisfactory compensation can be provided, inmates are driven by the idea that homosexuality represents the most accessible solution for carnal encounters with a fellow man. Society on the outside comes to the same conclusion, when it remains confined to the myth of the bar of soap picked up in the shower. In this sense, homophobia acts as a reassuring measure for those who are worried about homosexuality in prison.

The normative vision of society, nurtured by an institution designed to "re-norm"[131], qualifies as deviant, pathological and perverse anything that departs from a heterosexuality with a reproductive, affective or symbolic vocation for order. This norm, which is evolving in the outside world, is an essential reference point in a prison institution, which sees itself as a *repository of* cultural and societal *values*. Going against the grain of a "society built without norms (but not without

---

131. Cardon (Carole), *Ethnologie française*, Paris, PUF, January-March 2002, tome XXXII, p. 87.

principles)", as Alain Touraine puts it[132], prisons normalize because they fail to individualize.

The consequences of homophobia

The hatred of homosexuality is not insignificant in the economy of relations between inmates within the prison institution. Indeed, to avoid rape, extortion and other relations of domination, some homosexuals ask to be transferred to another establishment, in order to reconstitute a benevolent anonymity. Others are placed by the prison administration in solitary confinement or in units specifically for sexual minorities, to escape bullying whose physical and mental consequences leave lasting scars. Confinement accentuated by isolation, or confinement transposed by transfer, are the only remedies for escaping the terror that reigns around homosexuals in detention. This precautionary measure raises questions about the effects of discrimination within a republican institution like prison. This situation highlights the limits of the authority of a prison administration that has to isolate some, when it is unable to manage the criminal behavior of others. For homosexuals, this segregation has a victimization dimension, adding to the daily humiliation suffered by *conservatives of masculinity*. Because homophobia underpins mechanisms of violence, many inmates add the status of forgotten victim to that of recognized culprit.

The price of seronegativity

In their study on the relationship between sexuality and violence in prisons[133], Daniel Welzer-Lang, Lilian Mathieu and Mickaël Faure hypothesized that homophobia was an obstacle to AIDS prevention

---

132. TOURAINE (Alain), *Pourrons-nous vivre ensemble? égaux et différents*, Paris, Fayard, 1997, p. 181.
133. WELZER-LANG (Daniel), FAURE (Michaël), MATHIEU (Lilian), *op. cit.* p. 235.

in prisons. Ten years on, our interviews confirm this idea, and at the same time highlight the urgent need for action. In prisons, condoms are available in the infirmaries and in the *general store*[134]. In these two public places, the act of picking up a condom in full view of the public is tantamount to an admission of the prospect of sexual relations, which, with the exception of furloughed prisoners, can only take place between individuals of the same sex. The inmates we met noted that the condom basket is emptied every weekend eve. Invariably, their analysis leads them to conclude: "Some of them are going to have a good time!" But for every X inmates who accept the risk of braving the admission of homosexuality, how many continue to engage in sexual practices, more or less consensual, without any protection whatsoever?

In 1995, with a high proportion of drug users, the HIV prevalence rate in French prisons was seven times higher than in the general popu-lation[135]. The causal link between condom use and homosexual relations is so obvious that some people admit to preferring not to protect them-selves rather than run the risk of being labelled as *undesirable* or *deviant*. While aware of the risks of AIDS transmission, Augustin, a prisoner at Saint-Mihiel, admits: "I know there are some in the infirmary, but I'm

---

134. It is a storage facility for material goods, accessible to all and managed by inmates employed by the prison administration.

135. A joint report by the prison administration and the French Ministry of Health in 1998 showed that HIV prevalence in prisons was three to four times higher than on the outside. A June 2003 study (Ministry of Health), criticized from a methodological point of view (underestimation of HIV and hepatitis prevalence, as the ratio was calculated in relation to the overall prison population and not in relation to the number of tests car-ried out), reported an infection rate in the prison population of 1.04%. Internationally, a study presented at the Toronto AIDS conference in 2006 revealed that HIV infection rates ranged from 16% to 91.5% in seven Ukrainian prisons. Prisons are becoming "veri-table incubators" for HIV, due to unprotected homosexual relations, tattoos done under dubious hygienic conditions, and the use of used syringes (figures published by the De-partment of Statistics, Studies and Information Systems of the Ministries of Health and Social Affairs).

ashamed to take them. I'm afraid they'll know I fuck men. So, the sex I've had here has been without a condom."

However, a 1996 circular[136] states that condoms and lubricating gel must be made available to prisoners in the infirmaries. In reality, none of the centers visited had lubricating gel, the use of which is a conscious sign of sodomy. Some infirmaries have opted for the principle of sporadic distribution of condoms *on demand*. Prisoners are thus forced to verbalize their desire, with no regard for modesty. The limits of this restrictive conception of access to prophylaxis attest to a clear indifference to the risks incurred by the difficulty of using condoms in detention. This inertia is a reminder that day-to-day prison operations are suffocating under a host of *non-prioritizable* priorities. At the end of the day, the emphasis is mainly on issues of security and airtightness, seen as the foundation of the credibility of a punitive institution that is nothing if not authoritarian.

The foundations of the prison hierarchy

Sexuality in prison has a clear penal dimension. Prison homosexuality is posed in terms of standards of *right* and *wrong, acceptable* and *punishable*. To practice homosexuality is to break the code of honor of masculinity, to deserve punishment and to justify condemnation by degradation. Based on this conception, homophobia feeds an internal social hierarchy of confinement, the consequences of which are all the more important because they are irreversible. In the social hierarchy of the outside world, the *good* are free while the *bad* are locked up. This binary concept is reproduced in prison, where a stigmatizing hierarchy is reconstituted. Because men are always comforted by not being at the bottom of the hierarchy, a *culture of the worst* develops

---

136. Circulaire DGS/DH/DAP no 739 of December 5, 1996, article R. 711-14 of the French Public Health Code.

in prison, reproducing an intermediate hierarchy at every level of the general hierarchy. Among the outcasts incarcerated are *noble inmates* - political prisoners, bank robbers and kingpins - and *degraded inmates* - homosexuals and pointers. The representations that the kingpins build for themselves in prison sometimes correspond to the redemption of a reputation as submissive in society outside. Being dominant on the inside when you've been dominated on the outside - these may be the issues around which power relations are woven in prison. Among homosexuals, penetrators are held in higher esteem than penetrated men. And among pointers, adult rapists are more highly regarded than child rapists. The advantage of this pyramid structure is that it gives all submissives the power to dominate. Each inmate is therefore both submissive and dominant, according to the "there's always worse" rule. And because this hierarchy cannot be based on parameters of material possession, the *caste structure is* organized around questions of sexuality.

For fear of contagion, the social organization of detention is organized around an irreversible ostracism and division between men, those who remain men, and sub-humans, those who have degraded. The violence generated by this binary and irrevocable conception makes some people the *scapegoats of* others, and equates homosexuals with all forms of marginal sexuality, including sex offenders. Homophobic violence is a reminder that in prison, too, conceptions of good and evil, of what is *authorized* and what is *punishable*, exist as an echo of society on the outside, which judges offenders it relegates to prisons to punish them and prevent the contagion of evil. Homophobia reproduces in detention the mechanisms of punishment from the outside, and renews on the inside all the abuses of power identified and felt on the outside. Under the guise of a norm defended by the men's prison, power as a symbol of virility is a rule whose non-observance can give rise to all forms of punishment. Prison homophobia is a power to punish *evil* through the *male.* The radicalism of this stance is matched only by the sense of peril to virility in the experience of sexuality in prison.

Because homosexuals are considered subhuman, they can be used at will, to satisfy sexual desires on the one hand, but also to fulfill a whole range of interests, which can in some cases be akin to forms of slavery. Tolerance of those who cannot be eliminated is perceived in detention as a kind of mercy that deserves retribution. Leaving a sub-human alive, when political regimes have gone out of their way to exterminate them, is a bargaining chip that allows them to be objectified. Nothing belongs to them, least of all themselves. The human world does not recognize their right to integrity. They are therefore the ones who are primarily transformed into sexual objects, like beings who can be possessed, and who, in relationships of jealousy and ownership, are the object of claims and possession. Bruno, an inmate at Val-de-Reuil, comments: "Homophobia is very prevalent, including among administrative staff. The consequences are rejection, including physical rejection. It turns gay inmates into sex objects, so the rejected homo will offer his body in exchange for security."

Rape endorsed by homophobia

> "In many ways, the prison world is a parody of the outside world, and in this parody, sex is an essential element. Most pimps are convinced that in reality there is nothing homosexual about their behavior; they maintain that they are merely using a convenient receptacle that in more ways than one is preferable to abstinence or masturbation."[137]

The imperatives of masculine power are expressed in the ease with which weakness is denigrated, embodied in a variety of forms ranging

---

137. Jackson (Bruce), *Their prisons. Autobiographies de prisonniers et d'ex-détenus américains*, Paris, Plon, coll. "Terre humaine", 1975, p. 391.

from supposedly consensual, but conjuncturally imposed behavior such as prostitution, to submissive behavior such as rape. While sexual violence seems to be widespread in prisons, where population flows are uncontrollable, in detention centers, the *numerus clausus* and the length of sentences make these offenses more difficult and more formidable in terms of judicial or extra-judicial reprisals. Wolf, whom we met outside detention after spending many years in several prisons and several countries, puts the reality of prisoner rape into perspective: "When we talk about inter-prisoner rape, we exaggerate a bit. It exists, but we overestimate the cases, and it's like with paedophilia on the outside, since we've been talking about it, so we have the impression that it's increasing. In fact, it's never gone up, it's just now being made public."

Prison homosexuality is understood as a relationship of strength and defended interests, which often excludes any notion of affectivity in men. Thus, whether through prostitution or rape, the homosexual relationship that develops is schematically described as including a *weak* and a *powerful*. Under cover of the desire to inflict a correction, prison rape is paradoxically in many cases an argument invoked to requalify a rationally homosexual practice as an act of masculine bravery. The denial of the consent of the person being told he is a subhuman seems to be enough to disclaim any homosexual connotation in the violence committed.

Rape makes it impossible for the victim to defend herself or assert her authority. According to the profile defined unanimously during the interviews, the victim is invariably someone weak, and the perpetrator someone cowardly, physically strong or *psychologically disturbed*. Because it's common knowledge that the prison administration doesn't investigate all rape cases, and because confessing to being raped is tantamount to publicly signing one's weak status, rape becomes a form of intimidation that allows relationships to be maintained in the confidentiality of the prison *omerta.* Geronimo, whom we met in Val-de-Reuil, recounts: "When I was 17, I was raped in my cell by two Arabs who made my life miserable for a month. Abuse and barbaric acts, sodomy, fellatio. It all ended when I was released. The prison governor didn't want to do anything, he wanted to avoid getting into trouble with his superiors. Now I'm a danger to gays in prison: a simple hand on my thigh and I'd put out an eye. I'd even take pleasure in it, even if it meant doing more prison time."[138]

The law of silence, enforced by the threat of reprisals or the fear of being officially commodified by public recognition of victim status, is a brake on the trivialization of homosexual practices. It's a form of homophobia maintained by the perpetrators of rape, who intend to perpetuate their domination to ensure that their desires for penetration are satisfied discreetly. When it comes to rape, Bruce, a prisoner in Val-de-Reuil, explains that "the victim often hides". The power of omerta is on a par with the power of domination. Individuals degraded to the rank of subhuman, *subservient women*, keep quiet about what they know under threat of greater violence. Rape serves confidentiality, which in turn serves homosexual practices that are as indispensable to their perpetrators as they are impossible to accept. The accounts of detainee victims attest to the fact that homophobic violence is assimilated to the *desire for rape*, recognized as a sexual practice in its own right. The climate of violence specific to detention allows for a gradual and indefinite shift between homophobic motivations and libido per se. Paradoxically, the practice of homosexual rape is sometimes used to contradict a rumor of homosexuality. The weight of rumors is so strong in prison, that the redeeming value of individual reputations is achieved through extreme behavior, which denies the victim in order to reconstitute a self-image

---

138. Geronimo is 34 years old. He is detained in Val-de-Reuil.

within the group. Patrick Dils describes the power of rumors in prison as follows: "In prison, it can be freezing hot, and if the rumor is that it's freezing cold, everyone goes around wearing a hat and scarf. Rumor is always the strongest."[139]

The weight of homophobia is measured by the violence it engenders. Inmates have confessed to feeling devirilized by the realization that they could represent an object of arousal for men. The mere intention of a glance is experienced as an insult to virility. Yad, a prisoner at Saint-Mihiel, who says he is attracted to men as much as women, explains: "I fantasize about the bodies I see on TV, but I don't allow myself to look at them in the showers. Homophobia sometimes implies feeling attacked by homosexual desires, first and foremost those of others - which are the desires they express - but also their own desires - which are the desires they keep silent about.

The abuse of weak prisoners is seen as a symbol of power in detention. A power that is morally contested, but a power that impresses. Henry recounts: "A month ago, two youngsters jumped on a disabled man on pills. They're predators, they turn and wait...". This is the beginning of a relationship of possession that only comes to an end through the denunciation of men who can't defend themselves, which is seen as an act of weakness. Patrick Dils, a former convict who was released because he was finally found innocent, recounts his nightmare of sexual submission: "When I managed to regain my senses a little, I dragged myself to the sink and washed my face... I prayed that this would be the only defilement I had to endure... But, of course, I was kidding myself. The brute returned a few days later. And now he comes back often. Very often... Always at the same time in the evening. Sometimes he

---

139. DILS (Patrick), *Je voulais juste rentrer chez moi... Un innocent 15 ans en prison*, Paris, Michel Lafon, 2002, p. 126.

masturbates in front of me and makes me suck his cock. Sometimes, he sodomizes me... I live in constant terror of him entering my cell... Until the day when the ordeal ends, brutally. [...] Thanks to the determination of other victims, less weak than myself, I was finally freed from my torturers. Thank you to those who had the courage to speak out."[140]

In detention, violence represents the extra virility that enables homosexual sexuality to be requalified as the exaltation of a fantasized heterosexuality. Moreover, virility no longer depends on the body with which the phallus is used, but on the way it is used, and the intention of domination that governs it. Francis, incarcerated in Caen, remembers: "Men would come to me, we'd give each other blowjobs, but they always remained active." Penetration means oral or anal. In both cases, penetration with violence and domination doesn't necessarily make the penetrator a homosexual. On the other hand, penetration with tenderness and affection in a couple's relationship in detention represents the stigma of a homosexuality to be fought.

However, the virility that emanates from rape is not a universal value. The majority of inmates interviewed felt that the perpetrators of prison rape were cowards, inflicting double punishment on their fellow inmates. Rape is more reassuring for the perpetrator at the time of its commission. It's a narcissistic comfort, but this feeling of exalted virility only has a temporarily profitable effect in the alcove of the perpetrators' consciences. Reaffirmed in this way, virility can certainly be exalted in the collective, but the submission of a weakling is not such a rewarding reputation. In addition to the risk involved in boasting about an act that represents an offence, in prison rapists are also pointers. And in the prison hierarchy, pointers belong to the lowest caste.

---

140. DILS (Patrick), *op. cit.* p. 116.

Daniel Welzer-Lang points out that "contrary to myth and common sense, rape is not a gender phenomenon"[141]. In women's prisons, the motives for rape are certainly different, since they are not based on the defense of gender identity. However, even if accounts are rarer, the rape of women by women does occur in detention. The rarity of these episodes of violence does not exclude the fear they generate. Some of the women we met said they had been suspicious of the behavior of some of their fellow inmates when they first arrived in detention. In Bapaume, women supervisors and inmates revealed that sexual relations between women were subject to particularly violent forms of jealousy. Desire is a *matter of power* in male prisons, and a *matter of possession* in female prisons. The infidelities of some are avenged by others, and finally, as Dominique Lhuilier *et alii* concluded, "aggression belongs to both sexes, but they express it differently"[142].

The trade in bodies and favors

In prison, rape, prostitution and homophobia feed on each other in an interdependent way. Life in prison is a perfect embodiment of opportunities for transgression. Prostitution, for all its health and psychological dangers, is a material necessity, if not an inescapable indiscipline in the system of confinement. Prison claims to be a place of correction. In fact, it generates illegalisms that it is unable to pursue. The prison administration's position on prostitution is contradictory. What is seen or known must be punished, but the institution does not have the material resources to investigate and punish all offences. Loïc Wacquant refers to the tacit complicity of the prison administration: "It's an open secret among prison staff and workers that many inmates

---

141. WELZER-LANG (Daniel), *Le Viol au masculin*, Paris, L'Harmattan, coll. "Logiques sociales", 1988, p. 203.
142. LHUILIER (Dominique), RIDEL (Luc), SIMONPIETRI (Aldona), VEIL (Claude), *op. cit.* p. 112.

have to prostitute themselves to obtain the necessities of daily life, soap [...] not to mention education, which costs money and is beyond the financial reach of the inmates who need it most. In this case, the state is not content with depriving people of their freedom: it also forces them into material and moral misery."[143]

For men, prison homophobia forms the basis of a form of pimping in which the homophobic client becomes the owner of the prostitute, turning him or her into a homosexual. Prison prostitution establishes a sharing of roles and a hierarchy of sexual orientations. Because the prostitute is necessarily submissive, he represents the homosexual, the one who can be dominated, and the one who will need protection against homophobic violence. The *client* or beneficiary of prostitution services, on the other hand, is the dominator, the one who protects and possesses. In women's prisons, with the exception of rare episodes of racketeering, prostitution does not exist. Indeed, Nanou, an inmate at Bapaume, explains that "prostitution as such is a male invention". It's more a question of relationships of interest in a couple relationship, which resembles a form of "michetonnage", between a maintained, materially needy woman and another with generous material arguments.

Although it is not officially priced, prostitution, in its various forms, enables certain indigent inmates to obtain material goods in exchange for the use of an oral or anal orifice. In prison, everything costs more than outside. When inmates have no professional activity on the inside, the simple fact of wanting to smoke or make a phone call on the outside means they have to rent out their bodies, with only relative sexual satisfaction. Some manage to escape this vicious circle, managing their own financial needs and the rhythm of their *passes*. This is the case of

---

143. Wacquant (Loïc), *Les Prisons de la misère*, Paris, Raisons d'agir, 1999, p. 145.

Augustin, whom we met in Saint-Mihiel, himself a homosexual in his spare time, who has become accustomed to prostitution in the outside world, and who explains how prostitution works and what is at stake in detention: "I only prostituted myself for canteens. And then I ended up with a boyfriend in prison. On the outside, I was prostituting myself because of my money problems. It works here because there are no women. The clientele is often paedophiles, and mostly those with money. Prostitutes like me, on the other hand, are those who have no money and no family support. Here, only old people know about me. Those who have a vested interest in keeping their mouths shut so they can continue to benefit from my services."

The age of the *object possessed* is not without influence on the excitement produced and the pride derived from a relationship of domination. The homosexual market is dominated by young people. Augustin has no illusions: "I know you have to be young for it to work." They're the ones who get all the votes and around whom supply and demand are organized. There are several reasons for this choice. On the one hand, the young men are innocent and untrained in prison rules. Secondly, their *possession* by an older inmate is a symbol of strength and prowess. Finally, youth allows us to identify with the desired female body, through the quality of the skin, the suppleness of the body and the submissiveness of the personalities. In the end, the lack of heterosexual otherness is assuaged by age criteria, since it cannot be assuaged by gender criteria. In all cases, owning a man is a symbol of power. For the possessor, it's an expression of the protection he has the power to grant to the one he still sometimes refers to as the *bosom*[144].

---

144. The terms "giron" (or "girond") or "schbem" refer to passive homosexuals, those who allow themselves to be penetrated, those who belong to the most exploited category of individuals. These terms were used in prison jargon to refer to the roles of prohibited homosexuals in the 19th century. See O'Brien (Patricia), *op. cit.* p. 102.

Prison prostitution often begins with a rape, which stigmatizes and weakens the inmate, giving him a reputation as a homosexual and putting him at risk of being abused by other so-called kingpins. This first episode lays the foundations for a relationship of dependence and submission with the rapist, which, through violence and the denial of consent, marks the beginning of a relationship of interest with no way out in a place of confinement. This is how Alain Monnereau summed up his study carried out *in situ*: "A young, well-built, preferably 'primary' prisoner is placed in a cell with some 'old horse from back home', who is quick to lend him stamps, cigarettes and anything else the newcomer might need. The loans will continue in a friendly manner until the day when repayment is demanded, with threats and beatings, failing which the young man will only see his salvation in the offer to become a prostitute."[145] Finally, the situational analogies that bring rape and prostitution closer together are in line with Maurice Godelier's analyses[146], when he evokes the close conjunction between the notions of violence and consent. The only difference is that physical coercion is frequently absent from sexual practices in prison prostitution, which often represents institutionalized rape through a unilateral contract.

Concealment or the impossibility of being oneself

The obsession with concealing one's intimacy within a normative confinement feeds a sense of paranoia, avoidance and defensive behavior, more akin to perceiving society as a disorganized, individualistic jungle than to learning to respect otherness, understood as respect for the community. Given the risks involved in revealing homosexuality, a market in secrecy, underpinned by the fear of denunciation, is developing in detention. Homophobia instills a terror that can only be

---

145. MONNEREAU (Alain), *op. cit.* p. 46.
146. GODELIER (Maurice), *L'Idéel et le Matériel. Pensée, économies, sociétés*, Paris, Fayard, 1984.

assuaged by concealment. *Hiding one*'s sexual orientation is a source of blackmail, negotiation and transfers of interest, all of which encourage the creation of a place for oneself that is discreet but not too discreet, because discretion itself is suspect.

As in the outside world, individuals wishing to hide their sexual orientation resort to a whole range of stratagems. Embellishing, inventing, adopting attitudes and reasoning that are assumed to belong to a reassuring identity, are all self-denials imposed by the normalizing power of homophobia. This is the case, for example, when inmates tell us how they force themselves to behave in a masculine manner, to earn the approving gaze that constitutes a false complicity. Some even go so far as to buy themselves arousal aids, which they use only to *give the impression that* they belong with the men - by which they mean *the real, heterosexual men*. This is the case of Bruno, detained in Val-de-Reuil, who declares that he "pretends to borrow straight porn films".

Discussions of a sexual nature are as central in men's prisons as they are secondary in women's prisons. This *obligatory* passage is described as a form of hazing, a process of asserting one's virility according to heterosexual criteria. Silence and non-participation in this traditional detention episode are analyzed as suspicion or even an admission of homosexuality. Hippocampe, an inmate at Val-de-Reuil, admits: "Discussing sex is sometimes a must. I feel manipulated, but if you remain silent, you could be mistaken for a homo, or someone diffe-rent". It's customary to compensate for what's no longer practiced by a free and embellished narration of what was practiced in the past. Every participation in this kind of collective event involves the fantasy of being believed on the one hand, and the ultimate sensation of believing one's own lies on the other. This culture of lies is regularly referred to in speeches as "mytho". Through the importance of *appearances,* detention demonstrates all the *being* it does not allow. The discussion is intended to enhance and reassure a narcissistic image damaged by a non-existent, distorted or degrading relationship with otherness.

This ritual is reminiscent of the storytelling needs of teenagers in school, and the risk of being considered a virgin if you don't take part. Wolf isn't fooled: "People say stupid things to give themselves a profile, but it doesn't mean anything. It's either to make themselves look good, or because they're completely obsessed, but in fact they're hurting themselves for nothing." Discourse has a way of imprisoning realities that nobody believes in any more.

Chapter 2
Prison homosexuality

In prison, homosexuality raises questions and concerns. Often seen as a consequence of the deprivation of sexual relations and as the only choice on the horizon of long sentences, prison homosexuality calls for radical responses based on a binary and definitive conception: "You're either homosexual or you're not." This point of view is not without its anxieties for men who apprehend the slightest homosexual desire as a new, irreversible identity.

The mention of homosexuality in prisons challenges the principle of monosexual confinement, one of the side-effects of which is to encourage, or even generate, sexual practices that contradict the representations we make of a *population of invincibles*. In prison, the experience of homosexuality is the source of much confusion between the self and the heterosexual norm maintained collectively by the group. The prevailing discourse in the outside world has shifted from a presupposition that we didn't dare name, to a presumed reputation for generalized homosexuality, whose imprecise assessment reveals the distance maintained between the outside world and the punitive institution.

The question of the origin of homosexuality in prison is very prominent in the discourse of inmates, who wonder, for others and for themselves, about the sudden appearance in detention of sexual practices hitherto hushed up or avoided. The most irrational ideas circulate about a notion of *spontaneously generated* homosexuality, a principle which would make the prison administration responsible for sexual practices still recently considered deviant. Older and newer causal analyses of prison homosexuality alternately define two types of homosexuality, *circumstantial* or *substitutional,* suggesting a uniform explanation for manifestations of sexual orientation. The content of the stories we heard suggests that the answer is not so clear-cut, and that when it comes to sexual preferences, the binary vision of "I like it, I don't like it" proves imprecise.

Homosexuality is a terminology that is both *performative* in its stigmatization of beings, and *observant* in its description of practices. It is a sexual orientation that represents acts as much as it classifies individuals. In prison, homosexuality is represented as necessarily painful. The division of roles between penetrators and penetrated is summed up as "to *hurt* or to *be hurt*". Behind the questions raised by such practices, there is also the fear of discovering that pleasure and pain can be associated. This conception lends credence to the notion of degradation associated with homosexual relationships devoid of tenderness and affect, behind which lurks the fear of a return to animality.

Prison homosexuality throughout history

In all institutions, prisons, schools and the army, the authorities set out to flush out - and destroy - all forms of expression of homosexuality. Sexuality, in all its aspects, became the prey of predators of disorder, who built and organized institutions with the ever-growing illusion of being able to control desires through regulations. While Charles

Lucas[147] sought to combat onanism through collective confinement, Tocqueville advocated individual confinement as a remedy for homosexuality. In the end, between two evils, the administration chose to curb the worst: defeat homosexuality and take the risk of allowing onanism to flourish: "Solitary confinement for the night gave hope to the reformers, for the worst of 'unnatural vices' was thus avoided."[148] In spite of this, there was no stopping homosexual relations which, because they were no longer practised in the discretion of a cell, found their place of expression "even in the church and premises assigned to administration".[149]

It was only during the French Revolution that the idea of systematically separating men and women in prisons was considered for the first time, and at the same time prohibiting conjugal visits, which were often negotiable in the prisons of the monarchy. The penetration of Enlightenment rationality into the repressive institution made it possible to rethink prison in terms of the effectiveness of punishment. The aim of the institution was to promote self-control and self-discipline. Sexual asceticism was intended to help the inmate understand the personality failures that lead to offending. Prison became a total, normalizing and sanitizing institution. And yet, as early as the 19th century, some writers were questioning the wisdom of forbidding prisoners to have sexual relations, proposing that cabins be made available to allow prisoners to receive their spouses twice a week. As one prison governor elegantly put it: "While they're screwing each other, at least they're not sawing through the bars", sexuality appeared to the prison administration, like work, as a means of maintaining calm in detention.

---

147. Charles Lucas is one of the main theorists and reformers of French prisons, of which he was Inspector General in the 19th century.
148. O'BRIEN (Patricia), *op. cit.* p. 107.
149. O'BRIEN (Patricia), *ibid.*

Charles Perrier[150], in his study of criminals, relates the rigorous organization that could exist in French prisons with regard to homosexuality. A group of twenty "active pederasts"[151] had organized themselves in the form of an informal society, with a president, treasurer and secretary, with the aim of organizing the market of available *gironds* for requesting pederasts. Sexual services were priced with tobacco or alcohol, reminiscent of the monetary aspect of today's phone cards or cigarettes[152].

Occurrences of prison practices

Various studies seem to put the proportion of homosexuals serving long sentences at around 20%[153]. Others put the figure at around 50%[154]. Quantifying this figure is difficult, and depends on how homosexuality is defined. Admittedly, these figures are higher than the proportion identified in outside society. It is reasonable to conclude that confinement and the deprivation of the other gender lead to

---

150. PERRIER (Charles), *Les Criminels. Étude concernant 859 condamnés*, Paris, A. Maloine, 1905, tome II, pp. 199-200.

151. *Pederasts* are individuals who played the male role in homosexual relations. Their sexual behavior was justified by the circumstances of female deprivation, as opposed to *gironds* or *little Jesuses*, whose behavior was homosexual by instinct.

152. "In 1834, the director of the Clairvaux central prison claimed that 20% of prisoners from urban areas and 8% from the countryside became homosexuals inside the prison. O'BRIEN (Patricia), *op. cit.* p. 101.

153. "The only French statistics (based on a survey carried out in two prisons in 1983-1984) reveal that, out of four hundred and twenty-one inmates questioned, 21% claimed to have had homosexual relations while in prison (Monnereau, 1986). An American study (Wormser, 1983, 297-303), carried out in seventeen penitentiary centers, gave a rate of 30% of inmates revealing that they had had homosexual relations while in detention." RICORDEAU (Gwénola), "Enquête sur l'homosexualité et les violences sexuelles en détention", *Déviance et société*, vol. XVIII, no. 2, Geneva, June 2002, p. 241.

154. Professor Columbus Hopper writes in a study of sexual behavior and conjugal visitation at Parchman Prison (Mississippi) that "about 50% of inmates in the United States engage in homosexual practices". HOPPER (Columbus B.), *Sex in Prison, The Mississippi Experiment with Conjugal Visiting*, Baton Rouge, Louisiana State University, 1969, p. 5.

homosexual practices, which do not, however, necessarily requalify the sexual preferences of their perpetrators.

Generated and revealed homosexuality

The widespread idea is to accuse the penitentiary institution of generating forms of homosexuality. "Prison produces homosexuals", prison "makes inmates homosexuals". What's behind these accusations? E. Swinnen settles the question by evading it: "The question is not whether the prohibition of heterogeneous sexuality leads to homosexuality, but whether it does not arouse the desire for homosexual behavior that would not have arisen in freedom."[155] Certainly, the deprivation of sexual relations and the confinement of inmates in a monosexual universe are two factors that suggest sexual practices between men or between women. However, it's a misconception to believe that homosexuality becomes inescapable over the years in detention, when it's set up as an inescapable principle[156].

Given the highly subjective nature of sociological interviews on issues as intimate as sexuality, it is important to remain cautious when interpreting responses on the subject of homosexuality. However, unless we adopt a posture of denial in the face of the evidence of certain discourse and the sincerity of the interviewees, we cannot, under the pretext of intimacy, contest the authenticity of all the answers obtained. It must be admitted that lying by deed or omission is never gratuitous. It can be used to protect individuals from the wounds of the *ego*, or to protect oneself from the ravages of a terror

---

155. SWINNEN (E.), "La sexualité en prison, le régime de célibat en prison", *Bulletin de l'administration pénitentiaire belge*, Brussels, October-November 1981, p. 267.
156. "It is superficial to see the environment as a trigger for homosexuality, since the deprivation of women may lead to masturbation. [...] To clarify the debate, we need to take into account the actual pleasure derived from these practices". CORRAZE (Jacques), *L'Homosexualité*, Paris, PUF, coll. "Que sais-je?", 2000, p. 15.

that imposes silence. Conversely, we must also recognize that lies can be perfectly useless and therefore unused. So why should we not trust inmates who have declared that they have never thought about homosexuality during their years in detention, whose entire discourse remains homogeneous, harmonious and coherent, and whose behavior during interviews expressed no embarrassment?

Admitting that prisons *produce* homosexuals implies that, without any prohibition, and depending on circumstances, all human beings would indiscriminately practice both sexualities. This lends credence to the thesis of the psychic bisexuality[157] of human beings, as defined by Sigmund Freud and Wilhem Fliess. This thesis is not refuted here, but accepted in a balanced way, as a principle whose effects vary according to intensity. We need to clarify what we mean by the "homosexual factory". This power attributed to confinement would tend to demonstrate that we can intrinsically change the sexual orientation of each individual, by generating a change in sexual preferences through a studied process. This fantasy has long been nurtured by those with moral authority, whose need for normalization appealed to notions of "conjugal therapy". Yet neither electroshock therapy, nor individual therapy, nor chemical medication, nor behavioral therapy, nor lobotomies and other surgical practices, have been able to overcome homosexual desires. As in many phenomenological analyses, the search for the causality of homosexuality alternates between the innate and acquired debates. By analogy, this binary alternative of causality is reproduced in the qualification of prison homophobia. This question refers back to the differentiation between *homosexuality of substitution* and *homosexuality of circumstance*.

---

157. Psychoanalysis has given rise to an incessant debate on the biological or psychic nature of bisexuality. Sometimes conceived as the harmonious integration of the appreciation of both sexes, sometimes seen as the basis of neuroses, bisexuality is psychoanalytically understood as ontological and potentially pathological.

Typology of sexual orientations

Alain Monnereau speaks of "homosexuality through lack of choice"[158]. With the object of desire absent, inmates divert their arousal to an individual of the same sex. This is what most authors call *"substitution homosexuality"*. As the choice of women is ineffective, it is the substitute choice of men that enables the expression of carnal desire[159]. This view is shared by Daniel Welzer-Lang, Lilian Mathieu and Mickaël Faure, when they develop the *sexological hypothesis*[160].

Other authors speak of a "homosexuality of circumstances". These include Martine Schachtel[161], Anne-Marie Marchetti[162], Gwénola Ricordeau[163], Dominique Lhuilier and Claude Veil[164], to name but a few. However, analysis of the interviews leads us to devise a typology, aimed at clarifying or invalidating the definitions usually expressed. To see only surrogate sexuality is to ignore the potential presence of a degree of homosexuality in individuals who define themselves as heterosexual[165]. Similarly, to consider prison homosexuality solely from the angle of circumstantial sexuality is to impose the idea that we are all potentially attracted to both sexes, to the point of all having a more or less hidden desire to alternate sexual orientations according to confi-

---

158. MONNEREAU (Alain), *op. cit.* p. 36.

159. In the same vein, and from an ethological point of view, see MORRIS (Desmond), *De Naakte Aap*, Antwerp, Bruna en Zoon, 1968, pp. 95-96.

160. WELZER-LANG (Daniel), FAURE (Michaël), MATHIEU (Lilian), *op. cit.* p. 43.

161. SCHACHTEL (Martine), *Femmes en prison. Dans les coulisses de Fleury-Mérogis*, Paris, Albin Michel, 2000.

162. MARCHETTI (Anne-Marie), *op. cit.* p. 260.

163. RICORDEAU (Gwénola), *La Solidarité familiale à l'épreuve de l'incarcération. Une analyse comparative*, mission de recherche Droit et Justice, Paris, GIP, 2003, p. 147.

164. LHUILIER (Dominique), RIDEL (Luc), SIMONPIETRI (Aldona), VEIL (Claude), *op. cit.* pp. 66-67.

165. On the indeterminacy and indifferentiation of sexual orientations, see the work of Blumstein and Schartz, 1977, quoted in CORRAZE (Jacques), *op. cit.*, p. 11.

gurations of gender, space and time[166]. In order to understand the shift from heterosexual practices, which are often preferred, to homosexual practices, which are decried by the prison population, we need to define the occurrence of these changes, based on specific definitions and used here as a grid for reading the singularities of each individual.

Substitute sexuality refers to the sexual practice of replacing one gender with another, one sexual practice with another, while retaining the arousal and erotic construction of the substituted sexual orientation. Substitute sexuality aims to reproduce a preferred, or even exclusively appreciated, sexuality through an *ersatz* or substitute form. By analogy, substitute homosexuality would be like using aspartame to replace sugar. The desire is to obtain a sweet coffee, the gustatory expectation remains the sweet taste, but the pleasure is obtained from a diverted object. Substitute homosexuality exists only when heterosexuality is impossible. This homosexuality is a sign of *exceptional bisexuality*, in which the other person's body is accessory to the main fantasy desire. Tim, an inmate at Saint-Mihiel, sums up the homosexuality of substitution as follows: "By not seeing women, they change the way they look at men. Some get excited thinking about chicks, and practice on men."

Circumstantial sexuality is understood to mean sexual practice modified by its adaptation to circumstances, which raises the question of the alternating eroticization of one sex or another as circumstances dictate. Circumstantial homosexuality does not reproduce the attributes of heterosexuality; it replaces it. It's no longer a question of replacing sugar with aspartame; it's more a question of drinking tea when there's no or no longer any coffee. The homosexuality of circumstances exists

---

166. FRENCH (L.), "Prison Sexualization. Inmate Adaptation to "Psycho-sexual Stress"", *Corrective and Social Psychiatry and Journal of Behaviour Technology, Methods and Theory*, vol. XXV, no. 2, 1979, pp. 64-69.

whenever the subjective appreciation of circumstances recommends it (need for seduction, chance encounter, impossible heterosexuality, compensation for sentimental or sexual disappointment...). There are circumstances that remind us that homosexuality is not only possible, but also enjoyable. In short, it's *the occasion that makes the thief.* Marcus, whom we met in Val-de-Reuil, explains it this way: "It's true that I have a preference for women. Men were more for business [*nda*: porn], because I was short of money or sex." This homosexuality is a sign of *potential bisexuality*, whether recognized or not, as illustrated by Christian[167]: "It was on the way to the showers that I had this flash. He was undressing in front of me and I saw his ass. It was like a lightning bolt. No matter how hard I tried not to think about it too much, to turn my thoughts away from that guy's ass, it wasn't possible. [...] The first night we found ourselves in the same cell. We noticed our erections. I had relations with him for five months. When I got out of prison, I never wanted a man again, but I admit I got off on him."

An *exclusively heterosexual individual is someone who* defines himself as such, while lending credibility to his discourse through a benevolent tolerance[168] of homosexual behavior, testifying to a heterosexual orientation as an obvious preference and not a choice. The exclusively heterosexual individual may have tried homosexual practices, evoke them without restraint, and at the same time express that the attempt was unsuccessful in terms of the *desire to try again*. This is someone for whom the question is light enough to answer without embarrassment or aggression, that homosexuality is simply not attractive. By analogy, there are *individuals who are exclusively homosexual.* Such is the case

---

167. Christian, 38, married, testimony *in* Monnereau (Alain), *op. cit.* p. 107.
168. We saw earlier that any manifestation of intolerance towards homosexuality is suspected of being motivated by a hatred projected onto others of what one hates about oneself.

of Lily, a prisoner we met in Bapaume, who explains her attraction to women as follows: "I don't see what pleasure you can expect when there are no breasts!" The term "*exclusively*" should not refer to a scientifically exact and demonstrable mathematical quantification, but to a set of factors that give the definition a credibility objectified by enlightened subjectivity. For example, Ford, whom we met in Œrmingen, speaks with serenity about homosexuality: "My opinion on homosexuality hasn't changed with prison. I think I could stay here for twenty years, and I still wouldn't have tried it!"

Potential bisexuality means a *preferred sexual orientation* that does not exclude an *opposite sexual orientation*, without the occurrence of bisexuality being frequent or sought-after. Levis confides: "Today, I consider myself straight, but it's true that at one point in my life, I had nothing against going with a man, I felt bi." This is also the case for Nono, for whom bisexuality could only be envisaged by assuming alcoholic disinhibition: "When I was 14, at the young offenders' home, a guy sucked me off. We were drunk, and he was a crazy guy who tried everything. It was brief, but it's true that I got an erection, and then disgust too. I've since tried it with someone else... That was bogus too..."

Affirmed bisexuality is the unconditional shift from one sexual orientation to the other. The occurrences of bisexuality are not governed by a preference, but by a scale of possibilities that may also be linked to circumstances external to the subject (encounters, imperatives of discretion...) or linked to internal factors such as a fluctuating libido. Mulder, who met in Saint-Mihiel, puts a precise figure on his lovers and mistresses, and thinks that when he gets out, he'll go more with a man he met in prison and fell in love with: "I've had seventy men and seventeen women in my life. In fact, I'm in prison because of my last mistress... [...] I've always been with women, and had many lovers at the same time. That's just the way it is."

Generated homosexuality is understood to mean a sexual desire whose sudden existence is subject only to the event or sum of external events that generate it. This concept implies the negation of psychic bisexuality, as an intrinsic reality of individuals likely to be or to have been aroused by both sexes according to the circumstances or periods of their existence. Generated homosexuality assumes that it only exists from the generating fact, which can sometimes come from the discovery of a confusing and unprecedented situation. Fabrice, an inmate at Val-de-Reuil, remembers the promiscuity of the prison: "Sharing a cell gives rise to feelings, and I remember that desires began to emerge, no doubt because of the lack of sex. So, in the end, it's hard to tell the difference between feelings and urges."

Revealed homosexuality is understood to mean a latent and potential desire, which the circumstances of the institution are likely to bring suddenly to light. This concept assumes that, at more or less conscious moments of existence, homosexual desires may have emerged in an accessory or principal form. Revealed homosexuality is consistent with a principle of bisexuality intrinsic to the human species. This bisexuality is sometimes sufficiently latent that the occurrence of its revelation is never certifiable. Titi, whom we met at Saint-Mihiel, explains prison homosexuality as follows: "I think you have to be to become one! I'm sure they were already at least a little gay before entering prison."

What's true for men in prison is different for women. The fact that homosexuality is not a question of identity leaves a great deal of latitude for the expression of sexual orientations. Without calling into question the classifications between circumstantial or substitutional sexuality, women are more willing to change their sexual orientation, when circumstances allow or require. Similarly, when it comes to substitutionary sexuality, motivation stems more from disgust with the men they feel victimized by, than from consideration of the woman's body as a sexual object replacing the man's body. Dany, an inmate at Bapaume, explains homosexuality between women as follows: "Homosexual women in prison are often women who have been destroyed by men on the outside." The purpose of the substituted body is not as carnal as it is for men. It's more a search for tenderness and complicity, in which gender is undifferentiated. Finally, in female detention, the question of homosexuality is more akin to a question of *homoaffectivity*, in no way involving mechanisms of violence to defend the attributes of a gender.

Changes in sexual practices are also linked to the intensity of sexual needs to be satisfied. Individuals whose sexual needs can be cancelled out are unlikely to change their sexual orientation. On the other hand, unless they are exclusively heterosexual, inmates with a vital, non-substitutable sexual need will question their sexual orientation, reiterate a previous homosexual experience, or even adapt their sexual orientation through a substitution or circumstantial homosexuality, in order to satisfy the inescapable need for an imperative sexual relationship.

Finally, prisoners for whom the sexual need is circumstantially substitutable are those for whom the conflict will be the most disturbing. As homosexual practices do not respond to a compelling need for sexual practice, it is the individual's will and personal judgment that will determine the choice of practices, according to the equation: to resist is to be strong, to practice is to succumb, and therefore to degrade oneself.

Being and practices

The question of *being* defined by practices, or *being* independent of practices, remains unanswered. In the case of prison homosexuality, acts are recognized as performative, insofar as they suffice to categorize their perpetrators. Prison borrows the evaluations of homosexuality specific to the male gender community. *Being homosexual is* akin to a desire to perform sexual acts with a person deliberately chosen to be of the same sex as oneself. However, the motivation for these practices is not always described as the desire for the other as an individual of the same sex as oneself. Discourses distinguish between *homosexual practices* and *being homosexual*, according to subjective conceptions of variable geometry.

Heterosexuality between men: a male specialty

In male detention, the perception of others' homosexuality is particularly different from the qualification of one's own practices. When it comes to oneself, homosexual practices do not determine sexual orientation. When it comes to others, "to practice or have practiced is necessarily to be homosexual". This double standard underlines the danger of categorizing sexual orientation. What used to elicit indulgence on the outside suddenly becomes what motivates condemnation on the inside. Many of the inmates we meet have a personal history of homosexuality. These may include personal experiences in adolescence, or sexual abuse[169] suffered in childhood. Recounting collective masturbation at puberty was often accompanied by a detail, credible or not, tending to specify, as Ryan, detained at Saint-Mihiel: "At 12, we all masturbated together with the buddies, but each had his own sex!" Augustin also remembers: "With friends, we masturbated each other. It bothered me, because of my sex, which I think is too small."[170]

These representations of homosexuality based on memories of old, often experimental practices, have different consequences depending

---

169. Among inmates who mentioned homosexual practices while in prison, their discovery of homosexuality was the result of being touched or raped as a child. These events are often experienced as traumatic, not so much in terms of the sexual act itself, but rather because these wounds were never recognized by those around them. It's the denial of victimization that hurts, over and above the sexual act itself, often committed through mental manipulation rather than physical coercion.
170. Augustin, 21, is a prisoner at Saint-Mihiel and describes himself as bisexual.

on the memory each person has of them. The good memories attached to these "youthful nonsense" had the consequence of authorizing a benevolent tolerance of homosexuality, and even opened the door to occasional practices. Whereas a bad memory, often linked to the feeling of having been degraded, leads to a blockage and violent defensive reactions to the aggression represented by the homosexuality of fellow inmates. Armand, incarcerated in Val-de-Reuil for paedophile acts, remembers being raped as a child: "My mother never mentioned it again, but in the Japanese concentration camps, after being touched by an adult man, I once fainted in the rice sacks. Since then, I can't stand the smell of jute!"

The definition of homosexuality is left to the subjectivity of each individual. In the climate of great paranoia that prison provokes, and in doubt about the severity of others, it is therefore customary to keep such narratives quiet. This is the power of homophobia, the kind of homophobia that we agree to inflict on others, but also the kind of homophobia we fear falling victim to. Human relations in detention generate a form of constant terror, of which inmates are sometimes victims, sometimes culprits, and of which symbolic or asserted sexual reference is a central axis.

Roles that define practices

Homosexuality calls into question a person's sense of self, with the fear of not *being the same once* released. It's the fear of changing one's self-image through the loss of a symbolic virginity in response to the alternative "to have done it or not to have done it". It's also the fear of preferring tomorrow what we abhorred yesterday. To escape this anguish, men develop roles that determine their practices. The binary schema of humanity's separation into two genders ensures the survival of the heterosexual schema within the homosexual relationship: one makes the man and the other makes the woman. More vulgar, but nonetheless highly evocative of the judgment that follows, inmates speak of "fucker" and "cocksucker". In prison homosexual relationships, and unless we consider that there are also couples who are similar to the affective and libidinal union of two beings, the roles assigned to each person reflect a state of affairs, or are the result of a negotiation of interests.

Numerous terminologies distinguish the respective roles of partners in prison homosexuality. In Quebec, as in the U.S., the terms "wolves" and "serins" are used to designate penetrators and penetrated, respectively, in the context of so-called "situational" homosexuality[171]. Whatever the case, the most frequent configuration is to consider the man who *does the woman* as a homosexual, whatever the nature of his consent or the motivation behind his acceptance of sexual intercourse. Zizou, detained at Saint-Mihiel, associates this idea with the notions of religion and sin: "When we were kids, we were told that for a man, sin is to be penetrated." Submission is carnal before it is intellectual. Since the important thing for the man is to determine, by identifying the side of power, who carries the phallus, that's all it takes to qualify the relationship and the participants. This role is not to everyone's displeasure. In Caen, Francis, an openly homosexual prisoner for whom "being taken like a woman" represents the ultimate fantasy, says he imagines himself as a woman in the arms of the lover he met in detention. His fantasy is "[to] be penetrated under any

---

171. "Situational homosexuality" is a term developed by Helen M. Eigenberg to designate the homosexuality that comes with being incarcerated. This definition is similar to substitution homosexuality, although it borrows the situational aspect of circumstantial homosexuality. The reputation of the wolf, or active situational homosexual (considered heterosexual), depends on his power of possession and coercion. If he possesses a punk, i.e. a passive situational homosexual, he has more power than one who possesses a true homosexual. The situational homosexual's claim to heterosexuality comes at the price of this configuration. Other more or less nuanced terminologies are used to approach the phenomenon defined here as "situational homosexuality". Westwook refers to homosexuality as "occasional, acquired or optional".

---

circumstances", and he confesses to being particularly excited by the idea of abandoning his body to the entire disposal of other men. This paroxysmal representation of homosexuality symbolizes precisely the degradation that underpins and sustains the homophobia of his fellow inmates. The excitement Francis describes arises from his submission to the satisfaction of his lovers. His pleasure comes from his partners' objectification of his anus as an *indeterminate hole to be filled*. This is what Pierre Bourdieu distinguishes when he evokes the two faces of the human body, one being sexualized, the other asexual and therefore adaptable to the gender we wish to attribute to it[172]. The excitement he describes is reminiscent of Jean Genet's expression of desire in relation to prison homosexuality: "Jean Genet explained that rape is delicious, comparing the status of the raped man to that of the woman. Jean-Paul Sartre would echo these statements, writing that for Genet "the rump is the secret femininity of males"."[173]

However, because it's all a matter of subjective judgement between inmates, it's not enough to be penetrating to escape being classified as homosexual. It's also the circumstances surrounding the relationship that determine whether the sexual practice qualifies its perpetrator. A submissive relationship in which a kaid subdues a young prisoner, from whom he obtains sexual graces in exchange for protection against the hostility of detention, does not make the kaid a homosexual. It's more like a form of prostitution, a relationship of interests woven into a prison society organized around needs to be satisfied, and relationships of supply and demand. This homosexuality is clothed in the trappings of the heterosexual conception of the couple, in which the man dominates a woman seeking protection.

---

172. BOURDIEU (Pierre), *La Domination masculine*, Paris, Le Seuil, 1998, p. 56.
173. WELZER-LANG (Daniel), *op. cit.* p. 117.

The pleasure of being penetrated is not officially recognized for men. It's a deviant eroticism that *de facto* escapes the conception of virility and brings with it an ultimate representation of humiliation. It's as if it were a matter of consuming a forbidden treasure with moderation: biting the apple on one side without taking it off the tree, then turning it so that the missing piece cannot be seen. More theatrically, homosexual practices are unofficially authorized in prison, and can be summed up in the hypocritical tartuffery of "hide that breast I can't see"[174]. Men in prison have invented the practice of homosexuality without being homosexual. This specificity honors them, since they are powerful enough to impose the concept, in defiance of all rationality.

At the same time, identifying homosexuality only in the role of the penetrator is recognized as a slight interpretation. Indeed, for many inmates, in either sense, a same-sex relationship is one that unites two homosexual people. Stewart, a 19-year-old inmate at Œrmingen, explains: "I have gay friends, but that doesn't change anything. And what I know is that penetrating or penetrated, it's the same, in both cases, they're gay." On the other hand, finding a lover without resorting to violence sometimes means compromising on sexual practices. Prison homosexuality is often the subject of a contractual relationship, in which both actors, expecting the same thing, have to organize reciprocity in the sharing of roles. As Franck, an inmate at Val-de-Reuil, puts it: "Anyone who says he's straight and kisses, has a lot of homosexuality in him. The others don't kiss, they just behave like men, i.e. get sucked off and take someone." Indeed, it's often the impossibility of this tacit compromise that motivates relationships of violence and domination, in sexual satisfaction through rape.

---

174. *Tartuffe*, play in five acts by Molière, 1664.

The indelible power of confining words

In prison more than outside, words categorize, separate and distinguish, to the point of never abandoning questions of sexual orientation, however intimate, to the lightness of desire, banality and indifference. In theory, the inside indulges in a binary approach to sexual orientation. In practice, the singular evocations of the fluctuations of desire in detention contradict this divided vision of humanity. And while distinguishing between practices is a fact, deducing identity-based behaviors from them satisfies a desire to hierarchize human groups. In practice, the different terminologies and breakdowns of practices used, depending on the subject, give contrasting definitions of homosexuality. Here, the focus is on the words each inmate uses to designate the fact of being penetrated or penetrated during male homosexual coitus. The terminology used today by homosexuals on the outside boils down to the active/passive distinction. Both words are inspired by the vision of a balance of power between the dominated and the dominant. In the end, it's a watered-down way of referring to being a man or a woman. In both cases, words express a value judgment, in the sense of a category that *publicly accuses,* according to the etymology recalled by Bourdieu[175]. In prison, words impart an indelible identity. Gironds, or other "schbems", are bound to suffer the anathema of penetrating men, for whom the fact of being penetrated irrevocably equates to the loss of male status. Sodomy degrades in the sense of submission, while it can enhance in the sense of domination. There is a winner and a loser, and according to Geronimo, whom we met in Val-de-Reuil, "the one who penetrates is the one who feels good, and the one who is penetrated is the one who feels pain".

---

175. ERIBON (Didier) *et al, L'Homophobie. Comment la définir, comment la combattre,* Paris, Prochoix, 1999, p. 12.

Given the risk of being recognized as homosexual in prison, the qualification of the acts performed has a major influence on the answers
obtained. Is one homosexual as soon as one engages in homosexual
practices? Interviews and sexual experiences in prison show that being
homosexual, bisexual or heterosexual mainly corresponds to terminologies that confine. Rather than admitting without discussion the reality
of a biological bisexuality dear to the followers of Freud, here the *notion
of sexual preferences* is used, taking care not to fall into semiological
affiliations in which the detainees' discourse would not find itself. The
categorization of sexual orientations, however vague it may seem, cannot
serve the understanding of sexual orientations from the moment that
the conceptions *homo, bi, hetero*, have no objective coherence in matters
of identity, but on the contrary satisfy subjective appreciations, which
differ according to whether we are talking about ourselves or others.
The theory that "you are what you do" suffers from the inescapable
exception of those who practice or desire, in varying proportions and
according to singular motivations, alternating homosexuality and heterosexuality. The use of sexual categories only serves the authority of the
heterosexual norm, with the aim of reassurance, in the sense that not
feeling part of the *whole* amounts to the certainty of not being like that
other who worries or disgusts.

As in the society outside, tolerance of sexual orientation begins with
the need to name it in order to differentiate it. Outside as inside, when
it comes to tolerance, the *right to be different* - not to conform to the
norm - precedes the *right to indifference*, which renders null and void
any opportunity for discrimination. As long as the stigmatization of
homosexuality is justified in the men's prison, inmates will use this sexual
orientation as an argument for violence and domination. Tolerance is
never excluded, but it is often inspired by condescension, and assumes
in return that homosexuals respect the exclusive heterosexuality of
men who affirm themselves as such. Henry, an inmate at Val-de-Reuil,

explains: "Violence against gays is there to protect the world of men, and also so that everyone protects their own image."

Categorizing homosexuality as a perversion remains a contemporary credo. Being categorized as a *homosexual* quickly becomes a stigmatizing danger for the present and the future. To have been homosexual is still to be homosexual. And yet, if these words were not performative, some of the inmates we met would undoubtedly have practices with one sex or the other, without ever feeling identified with an orientation that exposes them to judgment. Having been so is also the fear of remaining so: stories circulate in prison of examples of inmates whose homosexuality, allegedly tested in prison, has become their priority sexual preference. Jason, an inmate at Saint-Mihiel, explains: "By not touching women, some get closer to men. In my opinion, when they get out, they'll continue to like men."

The disturbing compromise of bisexuality

Bisexuality is rarely recognized as a sexual orientation. The terminology is often overused to designate unassumed homosexuality. Contrary to Valérie Daoust's analysis[176] of this *undefined space* between genders and sexual orientations, the way people look at prison is based on reassuring binary markers. Anyone who is not exclusively heterosexual is easily labelled homosexual.

Bisexuality poses the problem of gender definitions for men whose gender identity has been weakened in advance. Landmarks built on questions of penetration and domination are turned upside down. Bisexuality offers a spectrum of freedom, the ability to alternate the

---

176. On the fluctuating space between genders in outsider society, and the definition of queer attitudes, see DAOUST (Valérie), *De la sexualité en démocratie. L'individu libre et ses espaces identitaires*, Paris, PUF, 2005, p. 173.

gender of one's partners in the same way as one wishes to alternate pleasures. It's also this latitude that makes bisexuality a worrying sexual behavior in prison, when it doesn't make people jealous. Bisexuals are perceived as "multi-prey" predators, and the temptation to have their power and freedom, when assumed, makes them *worrying* individuals. Prison walls seem to have been permeable to psychoanalytic discourse on the hypothesis of natural bisexuality in human beings. And in the end, the fact of not succumbing to it leaves certain phallus-holders with a feeling of incompleteness and cowardice.

Bisexuality contains an element of homosexuality that is all the more dangerous in that it is not exclusive, and destroys the implicit argument of a regulating homophobia. Inside more than outside, bisexuality represents a danger that could potentially contradict the heterosexual norm. Behind bisexuality lurks the fear of unfair competition between homosexuality and heterosexuality, from which homosexuality would emerge victorious. It's as if bisexuality represents the coital reproduction of the hermaphroditic fantasy: being the other sex while keeping one's own. This questioning is particularly exacerbated in male detention. The women, on the other hand, express no apprehension about this possible alternative. Moreover, in their homosexual relationships, gender roles are rarely reproduced or identified. Myriam, an inmate at Bapaume, says that between women, it's "the same role". Inmates seem freer to alternate their sexual orientations, and to consider going out with a man after having ostensibly spent several years with a woman in detention. For them, the variety of experiences generates neither fear of contagion, nor fear of indelible stigmatization.

What makes people fall for homosexuality

Depending on the sexual needs of each individual, but also on the temporal conception of sentence length perspectives, the question of homosexuality arises one day or another for most long-sentenced prisoners. Resisting homosexuality is often presented as a challenge that can only be met with strength of character.

Because the deprivation of the other gender weakens reference points in an anxiety-provoking way, the fear of homosexuality can be likened to the fear of a *revelation that* would contradict the established norm. What if the male gender community had the wrong sexual desires? Discovering homosexuality in prison is often akin to fantasizing about a *forbidden El Dorado* that would supplant natural practice. Discourses leave room for doubt about hypothetical homosexual desires, and relationships are rarely mentioned. This is the case, for example, of Lucien, an inmate at Val-de-Reuil, whose heterosexual life was disrupted when, for health reasons, medicine had to fit him with an artificial anus: "Maybe without an artificial anus, something would have happened with men." Lucien's entire discourse on the possibility of acting out with men in prison is peppered with hesitations, paradoxes and subtle, implicit evocations of regret. In the end, his sense of degradation is worse than that of recognized homosexuals, since he's not even fit to satisfy a man, which for him represents the height of being nothing. Similarly, Fabrice, an inmate at Val-de-Reuil, recalls homosexual desires born of sharing a cell with a fellow inmate: "I had impulses that would be homosexual by default, but I fought them. Sharing a cell gives rise to feelings, and desires began to emerge. With the problem of lack of sex, it's hard to tell the difference between feelings and urges."

The internal conflict between desires and prohibitions

In prison, there are those who have succumbed and those who have resisted. In all cases, the resistance is of a narcissistic nature, since it's a question of preserving one's self-image, reinforced by the presumed severity of a homophobic detention without indulgence. Franck, incarcerated in Val-de-Reuil, analyzes the factors that prevent him from *succumbing to* homosexual practices: "Ambient homophobia, loyalty to a spouse, the determination not to change in prison, not to do anything you would never do outside…".

There is a de facto inequality in people's ability to resist homosexuality. On the one hand, the intensity of each person's sexual needs has a considerable influence on their lability to sexual frustration. On the other hand, whether or not homosexuality was expressed prior to incarceration, means that each prisoner arrives in detention with a different apprehension of personal prohibition, depending on any previous homosexual practices[177]. Finally, paternal superego and cultural barriers, often represented by the emotional entourage, represent the most effective bulwark against committing what one would be unable to assume in front of people whose gaze is censorious.

Prison homosexuality gives rise to an often intractable internal conflict in men. They must either lose their symbolic power by agreeing to devalue their virility through homosexual acts, or make their power triumph by using their phallus in the body of a partner of the same sex. This dilemma is sometimes summed up in a consensual compromise, by adopting a heterosexual posture in a homosexual relationship. In his study of the concentration camp environment, Bruno Bettelheim identified the answer to this dilemma as follows: "What I do here and what happens to me doesn't matter. Here, anything goes, as long as it allows me to survive."[178] Isolation ends up allowing *self-deception*,

---

177. We've already mentioned the cases of inmates whose sexual orientation is said to be heterosexual, who have a marked preference for the opposite sex, yet who confess to homosexual practices, often as a form of initiation, during adolescence, or under the effect of cannabic or alcoholic intoxication.
178. BETTELHEIM (Bruno), *The Conscious Heart. Comment garder son autonomie et parvenir à l'accomplissement de soi dans une civilisation de masse*, Paris, Robert Laffont, coll. "Réponses", 1972, p. 147.

when confrontation with otherness no longer entails the imperative of conforming to a social group to which inmates no longer feel they belong. In this sense, the de-socializing power of the prison institution represents, in many cases, a *blank check* to succumb to the modification of a sexual orientation, or to various substitutive practices difficult to conceive of outside.

A homoerotic climate combined with carnal needs

> "This Michel who used to fantasize about buttocks in the showers, without ever having acted on it (he was a punk), on the way out, he'd tell me: "Me, I only like to fuck my girlfriends on all fours anymore, because I'm in the fantasy of boyfriend sodomy." Then one of his friends told him: "I'm not an object, an animal or a dog."[179]

Even if promiscuity seems to be adequately tolerated in detention centers where individual cell confinement is enforced, erotic imagery is deconstructed over the years, to be reconstructed from everyday visions of same-sex bodies. The weakness and weariness of virtual pornographic eroticism, combined with the lack of physical contact between bodies, generate desires to *touch* and *be touched that are* ultimately distinct from the question of gender. Everyday masturbation has its limits, insofar as the caressing hand remains one's own. There is no exchange of heat, no perception of odors, no sensation of touch. Only the otherness of a body can recreate the sensations of a carnal relationship that makes us feel that we exist through the existence that the other recognizes of us. This woman's body, which is so lacking, is sometimes replaced by a man's body, for reasons ranging from circumstantial homosexuality to substitution homosexuality. This phallus, no longer used in detention for anything other than micturition and solitary sexual pleasure,

---

179. Interview in Paris, January 22, 2006, with Jacques Lesage de La Haye, about an ex-convict in a psychology consultation.

is crying out for flesh to penetrate. The nudity of fellow inmates in the shower awakens a desire to touch flesh other than one's own, and to penetrate a human orifice, a desire that no artificial substitute can satisfy. It's the gradual emergence of hitherto repressed desires, at the heart of a homoerotic climate.

The palliative of the human body allows us to satisfy the animality of the *desire to mix flesh*. It's like releasing an over-compressed desire, *discharging* a contained libido, a source of psychic and physical tension. Touching, smelling and penetrating are all ways of satisfying the need to exult in one's own body. Homosexual practices in detention represent this need, inherent to the human species, to share physical intimacies that are part of the very experience of oneself as a man or a woman. It is the satisfaction of desires which, because they exist, and because they leave individuals unsatisfied, attest to the very condition of the human being[180]. Nevertheless, when the lack is disproportionate, when the feeling of completeness becomes an unattainable myth, sometimes irreversible disturbances attack the inmates' personal equilibrium, and durably disrupt the prospects of resocialization.

Of course, the libido remains attached to parameters of femininity, such as body shapes, curves, breasts, smells, make-up and voice. Even if the women most often seen in detention are female guards dressed in a particularly masculine[181] uniform, the satisfaction of the senses and the *ego*, when inmates imagine themselves remaining attractive, remains indispensable. Ford, whom we met at Œrmingen, explains: "As soon as there's a woman, I always think about seducing her. I always have

---

180. See RABOUIN (David), *Le Désir*, Paris, Flammarion, coll. "Corpus", 1997, p. 25.
181. There are no distinguishing marks to differentiate a female from a male warder, as the prison administration erases gender. The approach is identical, with the use of the same professional shoes, a sort of prison rangers.

doubts about how I can please, so here I have even more!" The erotic dimension of female guards was not the legislator's primary motivation when he chose to organize the mixed-gender guarding workforce. The presence of female guards in male prisons is primarily a response to the objective of gender non-discrimination in access to public service professions. Nonetheless, confrontation with female otherness is a not inconsiderable satisfaction in the experience of detention, and enables some men to bolster their *virility through* passive eroticism. This excitement sometimes takes obscene turns. As Angélique, a female warden at Val-de-Reuil, recounts: "When they know it's a female warden, they get naked on the bed, especially in summer, when the heat gives them a good excuse. They spot us by the smell. I open the eyecup and just check that they're not dead or injured.

The influence of sentence length on the lifting of prohibitions

As long as the way out remains within sight of an accessible horizon, resisting homosexuality is conceivable. On the other hand, the prospect of a distant release brings with it the fragility of a possible collapse of personal prohibitions. This argument is frequently used by inmates to explain the parameters that trigger homosexuality in prison. For Jason, whom we met in Val-de-Reuil, resistance wanes with the length of the sentence: "I've learned here that it's the years that make you practice homosexuality." So, for the *perpetrators,* whose assessable horizon remains drawn by the prison walls, acceptance of homosexual practices remains the only way to ensure the survival of a sexuality until the senses are appeased. It's true that a prisoner incarcerated at the age of 40, for a life sentence with a security period[182] of twenty-five years, is faced with the acceptance of being deprived of sexual relations for a quarter of a century. The hope of resuming a fulfilling sex life after the age of 65 is inoperative. Because the prohibition of sexual relations kills off

---

182. The security period is the incompressible length of the sentence.

the prospects of a sexuality for two, homosexuality becomes a palliative sexuality, of circumstance or substitution, which makes it possible not to kill off one's *sexual being at the same time as the* suspension of one's *social being* by the deprivation of liberty.

The study carried out by Hervé, a prisoner he met at the Caen detention center, on behalf of Alain Monnereau[183], seemed to show that homosexual practices took place during the first two years of detention, often on remand or in the remand centre, i.e. as soon as the presumed duration of deprivation was assessed. Excluding those for whom homosexuality is unthinkable in principle, inmates explain that the question of homosexuality arises in different terms, depending on the particularly distant prospect of release, and in consideration of the presumed age at release. A ten-year suspension of sexuality seems conceivable, while a twenty-year suspension is likened to definitive castration. Lucien, an inmate at Val-de-Reuil, explains: "Everyone wants to, but you have to stick it out. I'm not saying that after fifty years in prison... Right now, I think I'd do it."

Consideration of the influence of sentence length should not lead to homosexual practices being seen exclusively as a substitute for heterosexual coitus. The dimension of sexuality is never limited to the description of purely sexual satisfaction in the animal sense of the term. Sexuality must be understood as including all the forms of satisfaction it brings. It's about pleasure, domination, seduction, the feeling of existence through the existence that the partner recognizes. The evaluation of the lack to come and the potential to surpass imposed celibacy is based on the sexual question as the satisfaction of a pleasure that comes from bringing flesh together. In reality, the social and egotic dimension of

---

183. MONNEREAU (Alain), *op. cit.*

sexual relations is only subjectively apprehended through the conscious or unconscious consequences generated by the incompleteness of frustrated existences. Saturnin, a prisoner at Œrmingen, notes bitterly: "By dint of never sharing sex, you become an emotionless beast." The impact of duration underlines the idea that sexuality encompasses existential dimensions that go beyond notions of desire and pleasure, to embrace questions of identity whose resolution lies in the recognition of the place of the self, of the other, and in the emotional expression of the feeling of being alive[184].

184. LHUILIER (Dominique), "Intimité et sexualité des femmes incarcérées", *La Lettre du Genepi*, Paris, Genepi, September-November 2003, p. 19.

PART FOUR

THE LOVE LIFE IN DETENTION
- Controlled otherness -

"Sex is not love, it's just a territory that love appropriates."[185]

Sexual abstinence is not exclusive to prisons. Of course, there are individuals who are confronted with the phenomenon of lack, depending on their professional, geographical, personal, physiological or ideological circumstances. However, in prison, the deprivation of relationships is surrounded by a number of specific features that are not without effect on personalities. Abstinence is enforced, treated as an accessory punishment deducted from the main sentence. In practice, it is negotiable as part of a power relationship, underlining the subordination of some to the authority of others. In this sense, abstinence combined with duration is regressive.

In prison, the deprivation of sexual relations is at its most blatant in the visiting room, where it leaves behind a theoretical and regulatory concept to be staged as a condition of desire and fulfillment. Spatial and temporal contingencies, combined with the surveillance mechanism, underline the punitive dimension of external coercion, governing individual intimacy. This is the specificity of organized abstinence and controlled otherness.

---

185. KUNDERA (Milan), *Le Livre du rire et de l'oubli*, Paris, Gallimard, 1987.

Chapter 1
Restrictive conditions for love life in prison

"The experience of separation arouses anxiety; indeed, it is the source of all anxiety. [...] Therefore, to be separated means to be helpless, unable to grasp the world - objects and people - actively; it means that the world can invade me without it being in my power to react."[186]

In detention, visiting rooms represent a real decompression chamber between inside and outside. It's a place to meet *others,* whom the walls keep at a distance. It is also a confrontation with the principle of reality, which tends to fade with the length of sentences, consisting in remembering that the outside exists beyond a televisual virtuality and controlled epistolary or telephone communications[187]. Visits to the visiting room represent an axial moment for prisoners who benefit from them[188]: it's

---

186. FROMM (Erich), *The Art of Loving,* Paris, Desclée de Brouwer, 1995, p. 24.

187. Telephone communications with the outside world are regulated and monitored, and incoming and outgoing mail is read. Like any totalizing institution, the prison must control all kinds of flows that might break the insularity skilfully orchestrated by the outside world.

188. At the Val-de-Reuil detention center, the director estimates that sixty inmates out of four hundred regularly attend visiting hours (15-20% of inmates would benefit from regular visits). Most of the others receive neither telephone calls nor letters.

the moment of truth of a reality that is no longer dreamlike. Prison is de facto isolation, and some inmates are abandoned for the duration of their detention. This situation reveals a de facto inequality in the experience of incarceration. Of course, the prison administration can be blamed for the geographical *dispatch* it organizes, by moving prisoners to the farthest reaches of France, thereby limiting the possibility of visits by relatives. We also need to take into account the reality of prisoners whose family or friends have been dislocated by their conviction, particularly when the acts of which they are accused produce a sense of shame that individuals punish by "cutting ties". Finally, the material destitution of part of the prison population often reveals its emotional destitution. Some inmates even go so far as to claim that they prefer to live in the imposed community of confinement, with its host of reassuring carers, rather than the solitude of freedom, in the midst of society on the outside. Although frequent, these extreme situations represent a tiny percentage, which raises questions about the functioning of the outside world, making confinement more enviable than freedom for some. Such considerations underline a re-qualification of the prison, whose mission evolves between the officially disjointed functions of hospice, asylum and punitive relegation.

In prison rhetoric, the visiting room is personified: anonymously, *to have a visiting room* is to *have someone*. It's a place of affective exchange that enables each inmate to extricate himself from a totalizing universe, gradually experienced as an exclusive residual existence: "For me, a parlor is an opportunity to 'refuel' with affection and to rebalance myself, to find new motivation to fight. It's a short moment outside of time."[189]

---

189. AUZENET (Philippe), *Quand la justice nous casse*, Paris, Le Sarment/Fayard, 2001, p. 131.

Parlor problems

Beyond the eroticization of a context, the parlor in its current configuration poses the problem of how to measure emotional expression, while respecting the restraint built around a deliberately paradoxical device. Compared with the way things work in other countries, and despite recent developments, France is lagging behind in recognizing the right to privacy in detention. The "free" visiting room, as it is defined today, is a cheaply usurped term. Prisoners and their visitors are at the mercy of the supervisors' visual authority and disciplinary sanctions, which regularly punctuate behavioral disobedience. Even if the question of conjugal encounters has regularly arisen in the history of prison[190], until the end of the 20th century, visiting rooms were set up in such a way that physical contact could not take place. Encounters were somehow prevented by a separation device. In 1984, as part of the "detotalisation" of prisons when the left came to power"[191], Robert Badinter organized the abolition of separation devices. This political will to humanize prison brought with it a host of paradoxes that the prison administration has yet to resolve. For example, how can we manage the surge of desire when two people can touch each other physically, yet are forced to restrain the expression of a contained libido out of modesty or obedience? In sexual matters, the unsuitability of the prison environment creates the conditions for disobedience in terms of the legal article to which it refers in support of its prohibitions[192].

---

190. On the historical preoccupation with conjugal encounters in prisons, see RAMBOURG (Cécile), *Les Unités de visites familiales. Nouvelles pratiques, nouveaux liens*, Agen, Cirap, 2006, p. 7.
191. CARDON (Carole), "Relations conjugales en situation carcérale", *Ethnologie française*, "Intimités sous surveillance", no. 1, Paris, PUF, January-March 2002, p. 81.
192. Article D. 249-2 of the Code of Criminal Procedure. The Mémento du surveillant is more precise: "Sexual relations in the visiting room are forbidden during visits."

In some establishments, inmates have acquired tacit authorization to create a haven of discretion and modesty, to protect their intimacy from the gaze of the guards. Using whatever they can to obscure the view, inmates realize that "visibility is a trap"[193], and organize themselves behind coats, towels or sheets arranged as curtains around a table and two chairs. These makeshift arrangements are possible in prisons and other establishments where the solidarity of a large number of *long-sentenced* inmates has overcome disciplinary rules, under the authority of a benevolent management team. Even if the temptation to forbid these prerogatives is sometimes imagined when management changes, it becomes illusory to go back on such an acquired right. In an analysis of power relationships within the prison, Philippe Combessie noted the limits of a warden's power in the face of dynasties of supervisors and chiefs, but also in the face of the strength of numbers and the seniority of the inmates: "Every warden understands how dependent he is on those who have been there for a long time and will remain after him."[194]

Slow changes are underway. The intimate parlor, officially referred to in France as the "Family Visiting Unit" (UVF), is still a sporadic feature in prisons. After a long experimental phase in three detention centers[195], the French Minister of Justice announced the extension of the measure in a press release in June 2006[196]. In theory, France is in the process of equipping itself with the means to have a policy of maintaining family ties and sexuality possible for *long sentences*. In some countries, sexual

---

193. Foucault (Michel), *Surveiller et punir. Naissance de la prison*, op. cit. p. 202.
194. Combessie (Philippe), *Prisons des villes et des campagnes, op. cit.*, p. 162.
195. The first UVFs have been installed since 2003 (in line with a program introduced by the previous government) in the Rennes women's detention center (September 2003), then the Saint-Martin-de-Ré detention center (April 2004), and finally in the Poissy facility (December 2005).
196. Ministry of Justice press release, June 28, 2006.

visiting rooms have been installed within a few months, albeit in a less elaborate way than the UVF principle adopted in France. At the current rate of progress, it will take our democracy several decades to equip the prison estate. So, between intentions and inertia, the prison administration seems to be suffering from an incurable schizophrenia. We can't help but question this inertia. Everyone we met was asked to rationalize this state of affairs, which is surprising when it doesn't scandalize. This contradictory situation is seen as the expression of a disciplinary power that the prison administration no doubt has no intention of relinquishing in favor of a *fundamental right to inalienable access to sexuality*. It may also be seen as the expression of a form of indifference towards a population that is viewed with a certain contempt. Yet all the analyses seem to attest to the urgent need to modify the visiting room regime, in favor of attenuating the rupture between inside and outside. As criminologists Franck Danet and Sophie Ferrucci put it: "What is illegitimate is the despotic attitude of the prison, which takes advantage of its power of coercion to violate the principles that contributed to its creation. Our duty as criminologists is to point out that this remnant of totalitarianism plunges inmates into servitude, and places society at consequent risk of recidivism." [197]

To borrow from Michel Foucault's work, the experience of visiting rooms today is nothing other than the concrete, literal expression of the primary mission assigned to prison administration services. It's a question of *surveillance and punishment*, and the phenomenon of communicating vessels works in legal matters. Granting prerogatives to some means taking them away from others. Power over inmates' intimacy represents the subjugation of the individuals locked up in

---

197. Danet (François) and Ferrucci (Sophie), "Le projet de création d'"UVF" en prison verra-t-il le jour?", *Forensic*, nos. 7-8, Paris, September-December 2001, p. 58.

this "totalitarian" institution of "male guarding"[198], to use Erving Goffman's expression. Access to sexuality is representative of a demand for greater humanity. Charles, an inmate at Val-de-Reuil, reasons by analogy. For him, what is denied to humans in prisons is what is granted to animals in zoos: "The prohibition of sexual relations is something unbearable on an intellectual and psychological level. And perhaps even more so for their companions outside. In zoos, the animals all have a hiding place!"

The ban on conjugal relations in prison

The proportion of inmates concerned by the opportunity to meet a spouse during visits to the visiting room is relatively low[199]. As Franck, an inmate at Val-de-Reuil, explains: "I don't know if sexual relations are forbidden, what is forbidden is to show oneself! It's hypocritical, because here, it happens no matter what." The hypothesis here leads us to suppose that it's not so much sexuality, restrictively envisaged as a right or a possibility, that represents the inmates' main demand. Rather, it is the sometimes imperceptible effects of a sexuality that has been rejected and rendered impossible, or even transformed and controlled, that is verbalized in the "malaise" expressed. As Franck puts it: "The most difficult thing is that you can't take your time with your partner, so everything that has to do with tenderness, everything that makes you feel good with someone, without having sex, is impossible. Finally, these are all affective practices which have no direct sexual connotations, and which are part of a conjugated intimacy with a person understood as an object of desire.

---

198. GOFFMAN (Erving), *Asiles. Études sur la condition sociale des malades mentaux*, Paris, Éditions de Minuit, 1968, p. 11.
199. At Val-de-Reuil, for example, in 2007, out of 800 inmates, 443 received a visitor at least once.

A right that has never been acquired is more immune to claims than a right that has been withdrawn. It is tacitly recognized in France that sexuality is forbidden in prisons, even if the explanation is unknown, or even difficult to imagine. The deprivation of sexuality is deduced without rational explanation from the deprivation of freedom. It's almost a rule acquired in the collective unconscious by all individuals for whom prison is familiar. Ford, an inmate at Œrmingen, explains: "It comes from France's desire to punish more. Prison is there to punish, that's the system here. The same goes for comfort: why didn't we have toilets in the cells until 2005? All we had were toilets! On the other hand, when inmates in certain prisons have finally acquired the *customary right* to use sheets to hide the *spectacle of sex, and* thus isolate each visiting room cubicle from view, the prison administration cannot back down on pain of a presumed uncontrollable rebellion[200].

At the same time, the prison administration makes available condoms which, while not intended for homosexual practices in detention, are supposed to be used in the uncomfortable conditions of a sexuality stolen from the view of visiting room supervisors. And because the experience of detention is an added factor to the ordinary causes of impotence, medical staff acting independently of the prison administration are empowered to prescribe Viagra to inmates suffering from erectile dysfunction. Generally speaking, sexuality issues in prison are governed by a series of contradictions that underline the perversions of bureaucratic power in an administration that establishes its authority on the basis of almost immutable illogicalities.

---

200. This is also how the deputy director of the Caen detention center describes the management of this specific prerogative obtained by prisoners in Caen, to be able to reconstitute intimacy in their cells, during the daytime open regime.

Prisoners' discomfort

Prisoners see visiting rooms as a place where desires are irretrievably lost. The loss of freedom, freedom to come and go, pleasure and sexuality are all portions of life that cannot be made up for. That's why some people question the objectives pursued by legislators when they set up the current conditions of confinement. Levis, an inmate at Saint-Mihiel, points to a society's cold disinterest, which runs counter to any objective of rehabilitation: "It's because we're not interested in what's going on in the prisons. Invariably, the deprivation of sexual relations is seen as an extension of the deprivation of freedom. However, those whose criticism of the institution is more precise, see in this prohibition a clear abuse of power, seen as an injustice that undermines the credibility of the prison institution and fuels a feeling of hatred towards it: "Forbidding him to have sexual relations in perpetuity is one more sign, in D.'s eyes, [...] that 'justice is not justice', that it is only a sham, and that this sentence imposed on him is BARBARIAN."[201]

The problems raised by the sexual practices attempted in the shadow of a cubicle with half-height partitions are not limited to assaulting the view of the wardens or frustrating the inmates and their partners. Parlors are places where families and friends meet, and the intimacy they show raises the problem of tolerance of what some are willing to show, and what others are forced to see. This is the situation described by one inmate: "I saw a woman giving her boyfriend a blowjob in a normal visiting room. The guards see, the only thing they do is turn their eyes. But what shocked me was that my mother was next door."[202]

Prisoners' humiliation stems from the degradation they feel when those around them realize the lack of dignity with which they are

---

201. MARCHETTI (Anne-Marie), *op. cit.* p. 234.
202. WELZER-LANG (Daniel), FAURE (Michaël), MATHIEU (Lilian), *op. cit.* p. 101

confronted on a daily basis. For some, prison corresponds to a temporary insularity, which they prefer to avoid sharing with their outside existence, so as not to alter others' view of themselves as prisoners, not to confront otherness with the loss of self-esteem, and to keep the gaze of loved ones intact without the damage caused by confinement. Some are quick to declare that they would rather refuse visits than "impose the conditions of the visiting room on those around them". Henry, an inmate at Val-de-Reuil, explains: "I didn't want my girlfriend to come to the visiting room. We wrote to each other for five years, but we're not together anymore. I didn't want her to see me here, in these conditions, in front of all the others who often behave vulgarly, including visitors. I didn't want her to remember this image of me."

Children are also subjected to the same spectacle as adult visitors, since the playroom is often limited to a small space identified by a square of carpet. The way visiting rooms are currently run leads to *indecent assaults* that the prison administration cannot ignore. Given the importance of protecting children's privacy in a paradoxical and unmanageable situation, behavior is sometimes measured by the wardens, sometimes by the inmates. The spectacle of intimacy is permanent and generous for all concerned. Visiting rooms raise the question of the survival of privacy when it becomes a spectacle in spite of itself. Legal provisions and human rights advocate the authorization of sexual relations, understood as the consecration of the "right to respect for private and family life". As for the European Prison Rules[203], they advocate measures to enable conjugal relationships to be brought closer, with a view to rehabilitation, by maintaining family relations.

---

203. European Prison Rules, no. 24-4.

The love life in detention - controlled otherness -

In all cases, the intimacy obtained remains a humiliation for both the prisoners and their visitors. Meetings in the visiting room are seconds begged for, in the random tranquillity between two rounds of guards. The growing frustration of detention has had the effect of starving desires, and the satisfaction obtained is akin to the humiliation of the destitute, described by Saint Matthew[204]: "[...] the little dogs eat the crumbs that fall from their master's table". It can only be a matter of furtive sexual behavior lived under the continual fear of being seen and punished.

In the end, it's not so much the authority of surveillance that thwarts the desire for a carnal relationship, as the obligation to live within a single, watertight *gender community*[205]. The only answer to this problem would be to create mixed-gender prisons, as in Denmark or Spain[206], but this is relatively unfeasible as a general principle of incarceration, given the low proportion of women prisoners[207].

Supervisors' discomfort

The responsibility of prison guards is called into question at the slightest permissible laxity. On the one hand, their hierarchical supe-riors are obliged to enforce the extensive concept of an article of law that does not specifically prohibit sexual relations. On the other hand, by identification, some warders recognize the needs of inmates and the desires of their spouses, and do not particularly appreciate being

---

204. "Evangile selon saint Matthieu, chapter XV, verse 27, *La Bible de Jérusalem, op. cit.* p. 1492.

205. "It wasn't until the French Revolution that systematic separation of the sexes was considered for the first time." O'BRIEN (Patricia), *op. cit.* p. 70.

206. These include Aranjuez prison in Spain since 1998, and Ringe prison in Denmark since 1976.

207. In France, women prisoners represent only 4% of the total prison population, i.e. two thousand two hundred and seventy-nine as at February 1st, 2004. Statistics from the French Prison Administration.

transformed into guardians of modesty, any more than they wish to *hold the candle*, as spectators of relationships they sometimes envy. As Charles, an inmate at Val-de-Reuil, explains: "What's more, prison staff are sometimes made up of bachelors, who are embarrassed to see that we are accompanied by our loved ones."

Historically, the debate on sexual visiting rooms in French prisons has been distorted by the power of the warden unions[208]. Taken individually, or in the form of a questionnaire, the wardens, like Sigmund Freud concluding that "the recession of sexual possibilities results in an increase in aggressiveness", also admit that the deprivation of sexual relations is a factor in violence in detention[209]. At the same time, it is their hierarchical responsibility to comply with the application of the Code of Criminal Procedure in matters of modesty. Yet, collectively, the wardens defend the idea that it is not within their remit to supervise inmates' lovemaking. More or less happy expressions express the discontent of a profession with a poor reputation. Some fear they are "brothel keepers". Mockery circulates about "surveillants-Mrs Claude" or "Mr Durex"[210].

Ever since the project was launched in 1997, the majority unions have been *hostile to the introduction of* UVFs, while the minority unions have been *reluctant.* And while those involved in prison life generally deplore the same paradox, prison guards and inmates view the situation from different angles, and from opposing perspectives. And yet, identification between the two social groups represented by inmates and supervisors is far more common than either would like to admit. As

---

208. On the difficulties of changing the mindset of administrative staffsee FLEURY (Élisabeth), *Le Parisien*, Paris, May 9, 2003.
209. In the same vein, see SWINNEN (E.), *op. cit.* p. 279.
210. Durex is the trade name of a condom manufacturer.

Dominique Lhuilier puts it, in relation to the non-criminalized population, the prisoner "is both fundamentally similar and imperatively different"[211]. This connivance is built around the feeling of belonging to the same social group, that of the underprivileged crushed by a system whose general economics are not in their favor. It's not uncommon for a prisoner's family to include a warden, and vice-versa.

It's common knowledge that prison wardens are chosen out of spite, rather than out of professional or social interest. Interviews and questionnaires confirm this widespread belief. Philippe Combessie notes that, whereas in the past, uniforms were worn with pride even outside the workplace, today, even in rural areas, prison guards change back into civilian clothes before going home[212]. Since the abolition of the death penalty and the disappearance of executioners, the profession of prison warden has been one of the first to suffer the disdain of society at large. This is what Erving Goffman calls "stigma by contagion", which affects the social representation of the executor of "dirty deeds"[213]. The *egos of* each individual are enhanced by arguments of security, authority, protection and justice, which remain feverish in the economy of the prison institution, and which cannot be thwarted by any function in the supervision of frolics.

The prison administration seems to be held hostage by a regulation that forbids escape from the consequences of the paradoxes of prohibition. The entire authoritarian edifice is bound by the principle of accountability. If, whatever his or her position in the hierarchy, a prison officer takes liberties to relax the implementation of the ban, the consequences

---

211. Veil (Claude) and Lhuilier (Dominique), (ed.), *op. cit.*, p. 198.
212. Combessie (Philippe), *op. cit.* p. 59.
213. Goffman (Erving), *Stigmate. Les usages sociaux des handicaps*, Paris, Éditions de Minuit, coll. "Le Sens commun", 1975.

of a carefully measured and sometimes precisely negotiated laxity imply a professional responsibility that could jeopardize a career. Blind application of the rules also makes it possible to avoid all questions relating to the questioning of a situation that has been widely criticized, and to rule out solutions that are difficult to accept.

Generally speaking, the supervisors we met were not in favor of improving detention conditions for individuals whose deviations they were familiar with, and for whom a disgust was sometimes expressed depending on the type of offence committed. They do, however, express discomfort in their day-to-day management of the many paradoxes that put them at odds[214]. Since there are no longer any separation devices in the visiting rooms, it is clear that sexual relations have become all the more tempting as they become more feasible. The fact of surprising forbidden carnal closeness places the supervisors in the role of *censor of a ban* whose disobedience they understand. This rejection of an overly radical discourse on the application of the ban on sexual relations is also found in the discourse of prison wardens: "I've seen incorrect situations, I ask to correct the behaviour on the spot, and I have the power to write up an incident report in the event of a disciplinary fault. It's not up to me to give instructions to turn a blind eye.[215]

The supervisors we interviewed, while remaining firmly entrenched in their disciplinary role, are not overly strict with the prison population. The argument most frequently put forward to justify their zeal in enforcing the principle of prohibiting sexual relations in visiting rooms revolves around the most consensual of motivations, namely to protect the view of children present during visits. It's to avoid being at odds

---

214. Lhuilier (Dominique) and Aymard (Nadia), *L'Univers pénitentiaire. Du côté des surveillants de prison*, Paris, Desclée de Brouwer, coll. "Sociologie clinique", 1997, p. 74.
215. "Supervisor 5", met at the Saint-Mihiel center.

with this "situational paradigm"[216] defined by Dominique Lhuilier *et alii*, that their wish for change today is for clear, precise, unambiguous regulations to govern sexual behavior in prison institutions.

Prison officers are the "soldiers" of a system, and to make the *dirty work* easier to do, the mechanisms of power need to be clearly exposed, relationships of domination defined, and objectives officially stated. The legitimacy of the power to punish is never self-evident, which is also why wardens adapt the rigor of the ban on sexual relations in the visiting room, under cover of a mixture of compassion-identification and a well-understood interest in negotiating their authority. Given that today's visiting rooms are often described as "veritable brothels", it seems reasonable to deduce that leniency on the part of supervisors is very common after all.

---

216. Lhuilier (Dominique), Ridel (Luc), Simonpietri (Aldona), Veil (Claude), *op. cit.* pp. 105-106.

Chapter 2
The visiting rooms or Tantalus' torment

"Prison boils down to this dispossession, this depersonalization, this impossibility of satisfying a love whose obsession poisons the minds of all those deprived of it."[217]

The configuration of this privileged moment, where the inside meets the outside, is akin to the staging of *Tantalus' torment*. In detention, visiting hours are a stage for sexual frustration. Serge, who we met in Val-de-Reuil, ironizes: "Visits are like being given a glass of water and being asked to cross the desert without drinking it."

A man who has been deprived of sexual relations and carnal contact for months or even years is allowed to sit opposite a woman he desires. He has to curb his ardor, and sometimes that of his female visitor, to avoid the disciplinary sanction that would inevitably follow if the warden were to detect a suspicious rapprochement. In reality, depending on the configuration of the cubicles, *not seeing* is often tantamount to *not wanting to see*; each supervisor acts according to a personal appreciation of the notion of zeal.

---

217. CHANET (Laurence), "Prisons: du droit à la sensualité et à la tendresse... à la mixité", *Actes*, nos 45-46, Paris, June 1984, p. 52.

The construction of frustration

No doubt a religious conception of punishment is no stranger to maintaining a ban on sexual relations, in defiance of any ambition for rehabilitation. Psychoanalysts have taught us that desire, sometimes called *pulsion*, sometimes *libido*, is an expression of the life force. Dealing with desire also means dealing with the living. The planned thwarting of desire cannot be understood without the evocation of a metaphorical death, described by the feeling of *suspended existence* evoked by prisoners when they describe the time of incarceration. What Lacan called the "lack of being"[218]. Yak, an inmate at Saint-Mihiel, confesses: "I'm losing my humanity, I feel cold in front of everything." Daniel Gonin's viewpoint, after a long career as a mental and physical health practitioner in prison, is eloquent, both in his choice of words and in the metaphors he uses to take stock of the unspeakable: "Here, the stomach is hollowed out with ulcers. The skin is scabbed with eruptions. Sight is limited and blurred. But this place is neither an asylum nor a hospital: only prison has built such ruins. All senses are atrophied. Hearing survives only to listen for the clatter of captive keys. Many doors, little dialogue. Soon, 'sensory confinement' will have extinguished all perception. The only way to awaken this anaesthetized body is to prick it to the quick. Scarification and amputation are part of a horrific but vital ritual of self-mutilation. And if he doesn't sacrifice himself in this way, the prisoner has no option but to choose the solitary confines of a definitive prostration. In prison, the body is the last form of seclusion."[219]

It's hard to ignore the consequences of separation caused by the incarceration of a spouse. And yet, maintaining family ties is seen as a priority to help prisoners re-socialize on release, and avoid

---

218. Rabouin (David), *op. cit.* p. 77.
219. Gonin (Daniel), *op. cit.* p. 124.

de-socialization during incarceration. Here again, paradox reigns as a substitute for a response that the administration cannot express. The deprivation of sexual relations is frequently analyzed by inmates as a sacrifice imposed to make up for the offence committed. This is how Karim, an inmate at Val-de-Reuil, sees punishment: "When you're in prison, everything is forbidden, your rights are restricted, otherwise it wouldn't be a prison. That's what makes us feel punished for what we've done."

Prison as a *normalizing* institution. With the control of sexual relations, inmates feel that it also acts as a *moralizing* institution, albeit with some contemporary difficulties in sustaining the validity of its morality in a secular legal system. Frustration in the visiting room is experienced as a perverse sacrifice from the moment the object of desire is sufficiently accessible to be desired, and the authority of the institution sufficiently present to be potentially effective. Sometimes *primary*, sometimes *secondary*, according to Rosenzweig's test of frustrations[220], prison organizes sexual frustrations like a fast not unlike the Christian fast. It is through deprivation that salvation is purchased[221], and this mode of operation, found in many religions, is in this case appropriated by a secular republic, to the surprise of Marcus, an inmate at Val-de-Reuil: "It's a Catholic-inspired basis for punishment or revenge. It's bizarre in the land of human rights and in a secular country. It encourages disobedience, because deep down the ban isn't normal."

---

220. The Rosensweig test divides frustrations into primary and secondary. In "primary frustration", the object of appeasement is absent or even impossible. In "secondary frustration", the object of appeasement is prevented or delayed by a stress event. PICHOT (Pierre) and DANJON (Suzanne), *op. cit.* p. 2.
221. See also SABO (Don), KUPERS (Terry A.), LONDON (Willie), *Prison Masculinities*, translated from English by Arnaud Gaillard, Philadelphia, Temple University Press, 2001, p. 140.

This approach is supported by some of the inmates we met, who argue that there is a difference in treatment between "classic" offenders and "sex" offenders. Bank robbers, or classic offenders, feel they are being punished for something they did not commit. They often see the deprivation of sexual relations as a necessary, if perhaps counter-productive, punishment for the pointers, as much as unfair to themselves. These widely expressed opinions echo the penal construction of certain cultures. Punishment is thus seen as a physical constraint that owes its effectiveness as much as its legitimacy, by targeting the organ implicated in the offence. In the manner of "cut off the thief's hand", the prison institution must castrate individuals whose offence involves inappropriate or even abusive use of the sexual organs. This opinion reflects a pragmatic rather than ideological view of prison conditions. Prisoners refer to "common sense", without regard to the universalism of fundamental human rights. Their vision of fairness is practical and radical: prison is seen as an instrument of punishment, and another's fault is by definition always more punishable than one's own. However, Franck, detained in Val-de-Reuil for paedophile acts, tries to reason with a *different kind of common sense*: "*A priori,* for me, the best way to avoid re-offending is to find myself in a good sexual relationship with an adult. Justice should think along these lines.

Sexual practices in the visiting room: the intimacy of desire

According to the testimonies, the sexual practices carried out in the visiting rooms oscillate between the choice of foreplay, or the attempt at coital intercourse. The main criterion for choosing between these two practices is ease of concealment. Some find it easier to conceal the interlocking of bodies, while others find it easier to slide from harmless caresses to more elaborate erotic games. Tony, an inmate at Saint-Mihiel, explains: "I can't do without penetration. So we do it really fast, with no foreplay because we're too closely watched." In all cases, the sexual relationship experienced in the visiting room obeys a ritual closely linked to the circumstances of confinement. It's a sensual and/or conjugal reunion, in a public place, under the authoritarian domination of a rule embodied by the presence of a warden, and under the persistent threat of punishment. The evocation of this conjugal intimacy is that of the pleasure prisoners feel in existing. Their being exults in the rediscovered conjugation of bodies, with a person they appreciate, both physically and spiritually. Through kisses, the touch of skin enveloping living muscles, the desiring sex gives itself to the desired sex, the self becomes the prize of the other. This is the ecstasy of the carnal pleasure of the encounter. The same Tony declares: "It's a reciprocal request with my wife. I feel so much better afterwards. I feel really bad if I don't make love."

The binary operation of the visiting room

The circumstances of meetings in the visiting room reveal a binary operation between two opposing alternatives. This is as true for the inmates and the opposition they experience between pleasure and frustration, as it is for the supervisory staff, who oscillate between the awareness of seeing and the desire not to see everything. The situation in the visiting rooms is surreal when it constitutes the occurrence of what it forbids. This paradoxical regime has two main effects. It gives the illusion of a prison regime that is becoming more human, when in reality it consolidates the inescapable power of domination that *human parking* requires.

The pleasure/frustration tandem is made concrete by the removal of separating devices between visitor and *guest*. The encounter with the other is materialized by the touch of the body. The existence of the other becomes real, in the same way that for Saint Thomas, the certainty of the resurrection becomes acquired when the evidence is apprehensible by the senses: "If I don't stick my finger where the nails are, and if I don't stick my hand in his side, I won't believe."[222] Marcus,

---

222. "Évangile selon saint Jean, chapter XX, verse 25, *La Bible de Jérusalem, op. cit.* p. 1632.

an inmate at Val-de-Reuil, remembers separate visiting rooms: "When there was glass, the simple fact of being able to touch your fingertip was already great!"

Couples who meet in the visiting room know that pleasure will come at the price of the frustration that surrounds it, in terms of time availability, but also in terms of choice of practices. Because sexual fulfillment is complicated, prevented by the prevalence of surveillance over intimacy, some inmates reappropriate the image of themselves in the gaze of their partner, sublimating coital sexuality into a reassuring narcissism, in which the mirror of water is replaced by the gaze of the other: "D. looks forward to meeting his girlfriend in the visiting room so he can show off his turgid biceps, let her touch them, and witness her admiring comments. He's reassured: he's still a man! A real one!"[223]

In prison, pleasure is constantly accompanied by a prohibition, as if to remind us that any excess is synonymous with potential delinquency. Incarceration is primarily conceived as a suspended time during which the emptiness of existences and the control of pleasures serve the sanitizing objectives of an institution, in which sentences are served by purging individuals of the wholeness of their being for supposedly redemptive purposes. That's why the role of surveillance in visiting rooms is experienced as censorship, a reminder that punishment persists even when pleasure becomes accessible.

Frustration is seen as a sadistic, guilt-inducing punishment that signals the submission of beings to the prison, as if to remind us that punishment is all the more dissuasive for being continuous, persistent and totalizing, like the institution that organizes it. The paradoxical

---

223. Marchetti (Anne-Marie), *op. cit.* p. 234.

operation of the visiting rooms is part of these mechanisms of hidden authority, which, under the guise of bringing a little humanity into the prison, in reality establish an additional layer of domination through absolute control of prerogatives. The clandestinity of sexual relations in visiting rooms is both real and feigned, as is surveillance. Supervisors are not immune to these contradictions. Whatever they may sometimes claim, their surveillance function is deliberately not optimized. The technique that seems to prevail obeys the "I know but I don't know" rule. Unless they are in flagrante delicto, in a situation that could call into question their professional responsibility, the vast majority of supervisors let things happen that they are not *supposed to have seen*. The perversity of this approach lies in the fact that a disciplinary sanction can always be imposed, without the inmates ever being able to argue that the one caught in flagrante delicto is merely the tree that hides the forest of other disobediences.

In practice, the de facto ban on sexual relations in the visiting room only applies to a small proportion of inmates, those who will serve as an example. Depending on human relations in detention, the unequivocal application of the ban sometimes highlights the supervisor's desire to avenge his authority *a posteriori*. Given the surface area of the rooms containing the visiting booths, it would be illusory to think that any romps could escape a warden's vigilance. More often than not, disciplinary sanctions are not based on rigorous authority, but rather on the arbitrariness of a supervisor, who between zeal and laxity, asserts his power in a privileged human relationship, in which his position grants him the status of dominant. Supervisor no. 4 explains that his immediate reflex is to "inform [his] superiors. [I interrupt the report and inform the inmate that he will be reported". Supervisor no. 7 adopts a stance that his words convey in the form of intransigent, almost military authority: "It's forbidden, and must be stopped immediately!" The radicality of the ban insidiously contrasts with the gentleness of the sensations sought. Discipline punishes forbidden lovemaking with temporary bans from the visiting room, which serve to *set an example*. On both the warden's and inmate's sides, this binary is only mentioned unofficially and discreetly. Silence is convenient on both sides, since it's to everyone's advantage to conceal their respective disobedience.

Tranquility negotiations

Surveillance is described as being carried out at the *inmate's head*. Those who live their detention at a complete distance from the world of supervisors are also those who declare that they are "too afraid of being caught out". Levis, an inmate at Saint-Mihiel, says: "Over time, I've become very paranoid here. So I see hypocrisy everywhere." The freedom to engage in discreet sexual practices in exchange for denunciation or irreproachable behavior in detention makes some privileged to the detriment of others. This is the case for Xavier, who enjoys special consideration from the guards at the Val-de-Reuil detention center, thanks to the *heroism*[224] deduced from the offence he committed: "The guards are accomplices. You just have to choose your visiting hours carefully, and I always ask for a cubicle at the back. Then sexual relations become possible, but rather quickly all the same."

The power of the prison administration lies in its *knowledge*. And since social groups are relatively watertight in detention, in order to find out what's going on in the inmates' social group, supervisors some-times have to trade information for special benevolence in the face of forbidden behavior. In this sense, prison is no different from society on the outside, where the power of authority requires infiltration of social groups. Whether we call them *double agents, spies, informers* or even *collaborators*, the function is identical and the objectives similar. In all cases, it's a question of interfering between the authoritarian power of

---

224. Reminder: Xavier killed the pimp who wanted to prostitute his daughter.

some and the power of proximity of others. Prisons are no exception to this permeability of social groups, where the illusion of the rigidity of one group's power is mitigated by the impossible integrity of the others. These mechanisms are reminiscent of the "secondary adaptations"[225] described by Erving Goffman, which people develop to satisfy personal interests, quests for ease and serenity, and survival obligations. The principle being that every individual status derives from its singularity prerogatives distinct from those of others, and yet sometimes enviable for others. The power and freedom of each individual grows from the development of these prerogatives, which are bought or bartered in an institution where money is virtualized and possessions limited. Prison remains a society of exchange, in which everything material or immaterial has a price. While sexuality is often regarded as the only pleasure available to the poor in society outside, in prison everything has a price, and the gratuity of the outside world is sometimes translated into exorbitant values inside.

Relationships of interest are woven within the prison walls, increasing tensions between inmates and between inmates and warders. In this market, the relationship is fundamentally inequitable, and reproduces within the walls the inequalities of society outside, in defiance of the internal regulations that are supposed to position everyone in a single regime. Ultimately, the serenity acquired remains precarious, because in the event of a dispute, prison staff will prefer to protect their professional careers with the support of the disciplinary rule, in defiance of any prior unofficial commitment. In these negotiating relationships, the degradation of prisoners is at its height. Denunciation is the most widespread argument for acquiring the illusion of not being watched too closely in the visiting room. In many situations, especially where

---

225. GOFFMAN (Erving), *Asiles, Studies in the Social Condition of the Mentally Ill, op. cit.* p. 98.

sexuality is concerned, prison means satisfying individual interests to the detriment of collective interests.

As in the outside world, when it comes to basic needs - the very needs that the legislator, driven by politics, eventually converts into rights - the other is set against the self in an economy of survival. Thus, contrary to a democratic society based on living together[226], the experience of sexuality in detention often involves denying otherness by denying the interests of the other, whom we refuse to see as a fellow human being with equivalent vital needs. Instead of being an autonomous, personal and intimate activity, sexuality, understood as an adult practice, appears as a prerogative withdrawn by the institution and redeemed in detention at the price of de-socializing compromises. Sexuality is taken hostage, and the practice of it under uncertain conditions is a daily reminder, for many years to come, of the *permissions* that adolescents have to negotiate with their educators. Serge, a professional hold-up man detained in Val-de-Reuil, is not fooled by the negotiation of prohibitions: "In the visiting rooms, supervision is based on the inmate's head, meaning that everything is decided by behavior during the week. If you obey everything well, if you know how to cooperate with the supervisors when they need to know something, then you've got a small chance of having a good time during your visits."

It's also from these unequal human relationships that the prisoners will draw inspiration on their release. So many difficulties braved attest to the tenacity of a motivation to satisfy a need, the intensity of which varies between the vital non-substitutable sexual need and the circumstantial substitutable sexual need. In sexual matters, prison reminds

---

226. ARENDT (Hannah), *Condition of Modern Man*, Paris, Calmann-Lévy, 1983.

inmates that the satisfaction of personal expectations is achieved through transgression. These are the limits of repressive responses to the desire for order and obedience.

Practice conditions

The possibility of sexual practices in the visiting rooms is interdependent on the silence that surrounds them. One boast too many in the prison, and a prisoner can be *ratted out* by another, to the point of losing the benefits of the personal subterfuges that enabled him to defy the ban. The intimacy of sexual practices in the visiting rooms does not lie in visual intimacy, but rather in the necessary discretion that must surround each individual's disobedience. Before being the expression of a conjugated desire, the sexual relations practiced represent a defied prohibition, reminiscent of the educational authorities limiting the use of pleasures before adulthood. Thus, visiting rooms represent specific circumstances where pleasure is either the subject of total frustration, or the object of an anguish that some will find exciting. Depending on the sexual practices envisaged, forbidden lovers organize themselves materially to facilitate their lovemaking.

Consent put to the test by surveillance

> "I would have felt violated if I had to have sex at the prison."
> (Inmate's wife)[227]

As outside, the opportunity for sexual relations presupposes a compromise between the partners, based on their respective sexual desires and needs. The additional difficulty in detention lies in the fact that, beyond the simple question of the other's desire, acceptance of a sexual relationship implies acceptance of disobedience to the rules, of

---

227. *Ouest-France*, February 19, 2007.

the spatio-temporal conditions of lovemaking, of the presence of other inmates - in short, of all the contingencies of confinement surrounding carnal closeness, which are so many contrasts with intimacy as it is experienced outside. The visiting room is therefore a way of putting the partners' sexual desires to the test. This is all the more true given that the fear of disciplinary action means that the consequences of lovemaking must be overcome. As a result, many inmates who receive their spouses do not attempt or practice any form of sexuality; some because of their spouse's reluctance, others because of their own. Bruce, an inmate at Val-de-Reuil, explains: "I'll never have sex in a visiting room, because for me making love with a girl is clean, it's not done in a hurry, I take my time." Franck, an inmate at Val-de-Reuil, has had many sexual encounters in detention, but admits: "No, I can't even imagine doing that in the visiting room, the risk is too great". Karim, an inmate at Val-de-Reuil, felt more embarrassed than his partner: "She tended to forget that I'm in prison! She asked for too much, and I couldn't do more than I was doing. So it stopped, we don't see each other anymore, I prefer it."

The lack of privacy from supervisors and other visitors seems to contrast too sharply with everyone's sexual habits on the outside. Also, the necessarily furtive aspect of the sexual practices that can be carried out reduces sexuality to a hygienic or animal exercise, without arousal being built on seduction, synonymous with a rediscovery of the other. This is why, among the inmates who practice sexuality in the visiting rooms, there are schematically two different categories. On the one hand, those whose organization, and sometimes tacit complicity with supervisory staff, suggests a relative peace of mind for carnal encounters. On the other hand, there are those whose sexual needs are said to be vital and unsubstitutable, and for whom the meeting in the visiting room is often dictated exclusively by the sexual imperative. This is the case for Léon, an inmate at Val-de-Reuil: "In the visiting room, we caress each other every time, including fellatio and penetration. We try every time when partners come to see me. My concubine doesn't want to do it in front of the others. But I have other girlfriends who come to see me, and it's with them that I have sex."

If we go by everyone's accounts, we can conclude that there is a clear lack of information on the part of some, combined with an equally clear exaggeration on the part of others. Bruno, an inmate at Val-de-Reuil, describes the situation as follows: "The visiting rooms as they are designed, without curtains... I feel sorry for them. It's like being a whore on a Sunday night, and I also think of the anguish of being disturbed by a warden." In reality, this contrast in discourse also reveals a lack of precision in everyone's vision of sexual behavior. Anything other than penetration or oral sex is excluded from the definition of sexuality. And yet, without going as far as the culmination of these practices, conjugal encounters in the visiting room are privileged moments for secondary forms of sexuality, expressed through positions, touching, closeness and kissing. In the end, whatever happens, unless the moment of the visit has been the object of a conflict, the inmates claim to return to their cells "so much better", after having had a sexual relationship in the visiting room. The week that follows seems lighter and the experience of detention more relaxed. Roland Agret narrates this new-found pleni-tude: "So Virginie goes to the visiting room with a pair of torn tights between her legs under a long skirt. On the sly, watching the guard's comings and goings, she offers Paul her sex. He plunges himself into it. A few moments that give him a kind of eternity of happiness."[228]

In the visiting room, there are those who dare and those who don't. Daring does not necessarily mean reaching orgasm at the moment of

---

228. AGRET (Roland), *L'Amour enchristé. Lettre ouverte à Élisabeth Guigou, garde des Sceaux et ministre de la Justice*, Paris, Blanche, 1998, p. 117.

The love life in detention - controlled otherness -

the encounter. Sometimes, it's enough to create new excitements in an erotic construction elaborated for two, only to meet again at a distance, in a virtual meeting at a precise time, in the schizophrenia of two distinct places. This is the case for Sly, a prisoner at Œrmingen, when he talks about his restrained yet effective practices: "We have incredible desire in the visiting room. All we do is touch each other through our clothes, because of the warders. We both get erections, and sometimes I can make her come like this through her clothes. We leave in a state that's unbelievable. She masturbates when she leaves for her hotel, and so do I. She wasn't the type to do that."

Sexuality appears to be a way of *rediscovering the* other, understood as a substitute for the solitude of imprisonment, but also a way of rediscovering oneself as an actor in the pleasure, seduction and feelings of the other. In both cases, sexual practices in the visiting room are experienced as reassuring by those who choose to indulge in them. Others, on the other hand, see this intersection between the worlds of outside and inside as too mortifying a moment, to the point of concluding that it's better not to have a visitor, rather than endure the frustration and separation followed by the return to the solitude of the cell.

Clandestinity and symbolic castration

"They were kissing like starving men."[229]

In the visiting rooms, poorly managed secrecy means immediate censorship of pleasure. Male inmates are subjected to the guards, in front of their spouses who witness their sense of diminishment. This situation is experienced as a degradation of their status as males; they are stripped of their legitimacy to give pleasure and satisfy their partner's desire. Women, whether inmates or companions of inmates, are not

---

229. LAMBERT (Christophe), *Derrière les barreaux*, Paris, Michalon, 1999, p. 30.

spared the lack of dignity offered by visiting rooms in their current configuration. They also experience this degradation through the public display of their intimacy. They say they are "discovered" in their sexual activity, taken at fault by the warders as if they were indulging in a *sexuality of interest* like prostitutes.

The fact of being interrupted in an embrace by guards enforcing the rules is akin to a castration scene in which the spouse is a privileged witness. It's a public questioning of intimate behavior, and underlines the submission of couples to the authority of the prison administration. The current situation in the visiting rooms is not only humiliating because of the shamelessness it provokes, but also because of the intrusion of an authority into a couple's relationship in which the two actors are no longer the only ones to decide. The conjugal encounter, organized in this way, loses the spontaneity that makes up human relations in the outside world, and is carried out according to artifices that interfere with the question of desire. Parlors remain staged events in which individuals seek to rediscover *naturalness* in a situation that is definitely not natural.

The sword of Damocles hanging over attempted lovemaking is not only the fear of disciplinary action[230]. From the point of view of self-esteem and self-worth, it appears from the speeches heard that the leniency of the wardens is also equated with a feeling of submission: it is in fact at the moment when the despot pardons his victim that the latter is most submissive to him. Submission is often born of the recognition or implicit negotiation engendered by a hierarchical relationship. "It's

---

230. When inmates are caught in flagrante delicto of a sexual relationship, the supervisors draw up a report which is forwarded to the management, who take a decision based on the circumstances and any recurrence of the offence, prohibiting visits to the visiting room for a given period. The penalty for an attempt at sexual rapprochement is therefore a total ban on conjugal visits to the visiting room.

for the pardon I've been given that I'll continue to submit", and in the end, whether lenient or severe, the prison administration's authority over inmates' sexual behavior remains arbitrary, and therefore potentially discriminatory. Whether forbidden or permitted, from the moment a behavior is authorized by a third party, it escapes the free will of the person concerned. While there are couples whose relationship is sufficiently solidified on the outside to withstand the constraints of *conjugal relations for the duration of* their incarceration, there are also a certain number of inmates for whom visiting room conditions rule out any possibility of carnal relations. This is the case, for example, of Béa, an inmate at Bapaume, who remarried in prison to an inmate she met on the other side of the men's wall: "Even on our wedding day here in Bapaume, we didn't have a single moment of intimacy. So of course I love him, and that's what keeps me going, but I'm not sure I'm optimistic about getting out... I'm a bit scared, given that I only know him for an hour a week, with a table between the two of us, and a warden wandering around."

Sometimes it's the wives who feel it's impossible to indulge in such furtive, risky relationships. Sometimes it's the men who can't find anything to get excited about in the circumstances, or to reassure their masculine power. Paradoxically, some inmates also admit that the fear of being caught out sometimes combines with the excitement that comes with defying the forbidden. This excitement can also be shared by the partner, or even aroused by her. As Jason, an inmate at Val-de-Reuil, recounts: "She often asked me how I was doing sexually in prison. She was much more excited about it than I was. A lot of inmates say that their wives are excited about coming to prison and having sex in the visiting room."

One of the markers that incarceration can break is the reversal of relationships of dependence and authority. The visiting room depicts the dependence of a man waiting for a woman on the move. The man is visited in the same way as a person who is diminished, ill, without autonomy. He finds himself dependent on the outside world, to which he no longer has access. It's the woman who gives and the man who receives. Symbolically, this posture contradicts the sexual power inferred from the ability to penetrate, to give one's sex to one's partner. This is also Erich Fromm's conclusion when he says: "Male sexuality reaches its climax in the act of giving; the man gives himself, his sexual organ, to the woman. At the moment of orgasm, he gives her his seed. He can't avoid giving if he's powerful. If he can't give, he's impotent."[231]

Prison provokes this symbolic castration in men, who struggle to regain their status as dominant, hard-driving males in the degrading circumstances of the visiting room. The disruption of self-esteem frequently leads to self-rejection, which some inmates metaphorize in self-mutilation. Others prefer to cease all relationships and refuse all visits to escape this regular staging of what they see as their decline. Roles are also disrupted for imprisoned mothers, who lose their status as protective mother in favor of a spouse on the loose or any other educator. These disruptions to gender roles are not without effect on the sexual functioning of individuals. Some women report that their menstruation disappears while they are in prison. Because cultural gender markers are overturned, confinement alters self-esteem to the point of leaving individuals bereft of their sense of existence within the group. The visiting room, as it is constituted, reveals inmates' dependence on the outside world, and underlines the degradation of their status as men and women. The challenge of the Family Visiting Units is to reconstitute, over time and in a chosen space, the conditions of a conjugal and social status, in which prisoners regain their conjugal

---

231. Fromm (Erich), *op. cit.* p. 40.

reference points, their self-esteem, and consequently, at a sexual level, their respective positions as men and women.

The premeditated staging of fantasies

To thwart the conditions of Tantalus' torment, lovers prepare their encounters. It's a question of devising appropriate clothing to allow quick access to each other's bodies. It's also a question of compensating for daily seduction by concentrating on the artifice of a unique encounter in a limited time and space. Dressing for the occasion can be a source of excitement.

The men wear jogging pants, without belts, buttons or zippers to open. This facilitates access to the genitals, while the maneuvers required to avoid punishment are carried out more quickly. As for the women, they wear loose-fitting coats whose primary purpose is to act as curtains or screens. They also wear full skirts to conceal the entanglement of their bodies when the lovers decide on seated penetration.

The most discreet relations are those involving the hands of one person on the body of the other. The ambiguity of the situation stems from the fact that, since the prohibition of sexual relations is justified only by the need to respect modesty, two bodies are supposed to be able to modestly approach each other, provided that the interlocking of the sexes is concealed by fabric. The power of the prison administration intervenes between the lovers, censoring a relationship that is too fused. In the words of Max, an inmate at Œrmingen, we see the indispensable complicity of the spouse, the latitude given by the wardens in their zeal to monitor, and the devices put in place to facilitate the realization of the carnal relationship: "It happens when we need it. I ask for an extension to the visiting room, so the families go out for a quarter of an hour before the others arrive. If we're discreet, we can even go as far as penetration. She puts on a full skirt and a big sweater to cover it up.

So we always do it sitting down. It usually lasts between ten and thirty minutes, depending on whether the supervisor gets up or not. She's also very scared we'll get caught, but she needs it too."

In this case, because visiting rooms are also places for family reunions, lovers often have to choose between the importance of conjugal reunions and the importance of filial reunions. If the partner is accompanied by children, given the configuration of the visiting rooms, and unless she puts on an immodest show, sexuality will be excluded.

The problems posed by sexuality in detention differ depending on whether the prisoners are women or men. The prison administration does not intend to have to deal with the situation of "baby visiting rooms"[232]. So, contrary to the theory on the "euphemization of the prison"[233] developed by Dominique Lhuilier *et alii*, the discipline of visiting hours in women's prisons is quite specific. Granting women prisoners sexuality means taking the risk of them becoming pregnant. Doudou, an inmate at Val-de-Reuil, sees this as justification for banning sexual relations in male prison visiting rooms. For him, it's an argument of gender equality: "How can sexuality be granted to male prisoners and not to women? The problem with women's prisons is that the administration has no desire to have pregnant inmates." Despite this, and despite the fact that the visiting rooms at Bapaume are cubicles closed by glass doors, with an immovable table, Nanou sometimes manages to escape the inquisitive gaze of the warders, to allow herself what she was unable to do on her wedding day in detention: "At Christmas in the visiting room, I thought I was frigid, in fact I asked for more. It's the shame of girls. [...] He's very keen too.

---

232. CARDON (Carole), *op. cit.* p. 86.
233. LHUILIER (Dominique), RIDEL (Luc), SIMONPIETRI (Aldona), VEIL (Claude), *op. cit.* p. 252.

The matron thinks my clothes are indecent. But I wear skirts in the visiting room."

Concern for privacy: seeing and being seen

In a stifled universe of potential surveillance, stares, eavesdropping, suspected odors and body searches, the stakes of the conjugal encounter, beyond society's representation of intimacy from the outside, exacerbate the imperatives of the need to be *hidden*. The principle of guarded confinement leads to a fragmentation of awareness of the singular in its relationship with otherness. The individual is never alone with the other, because the encounter is always accompanied by the collective in which the curiosity of visual and auditory surveillance is embedded. And yet, for each prisoner, a visit to the visiting room represents a suspended moment in which to find oneself before being able to find the other. To ensure that this encounter gives the impression of having been experienced, the challenge is to create conditions that give the inmate the illusion of a reality in which he or she is the *sole actor in* his or her own existence. Yet it is undoubtedly in the visiting room, during this privileged moment of encounter between outside and inside, that Jeremy Bentham's *Panopticon*[234] is best embodied. Prisoners and their visitors will therefore attempt to thwart the *rules of seeing,* of which the wardens remain the masters, out of resistance to the certainty that Charles, an inmate at Val-de-Reuil, expresses: "At no time can you say 'nobody's looking at me'!"

---

234. An eighteenth-century British jurist and philosopher, Jeremy Bentham developed the doctrine of "utilitarianism", which states that individuals are essentially driven by the interests of pleasure and the management of punishment. He created the concept of the *panoptic*, a kind of model prison based on permanent observation of inmates' movements, from a central point allowing a global view of the cells: "to be seen without seeing". The panoptic process is based on a particular architecture, obeying a principle of continual surveillance that Michel Foucault was to criticize and find in other forms of social construction, such as factories and schools.

Intimacy melted into the collective

The space devoted to meetings in visiting rooms is particularly symptomatic of the administration's desire to blend intimacy into the collective. In most prisons, visiting rooms are common rooms divided by half-height cubicles, open on one side, and sometimes shared by two inmates. When intimacy is not disturbed by the gaze of the guards, the view and hearing of relations in the visiting room are shared by all the other inmates and their visitors. The geographical and architectural configuration of the visiting rooms is a clear denial of both visual and auditory privacy. Marital encounters in the visiting rooms can be likened to scenes of exhibition of affection as much as of sexuality. After a daily routine that inmates describe as "infantilizing and mothering", Tom, an inmate at Œrmingen, explains: "We unlearn how to live, we're assisted, and when we get out, I suppose it's hard to regain autonomy." So, in addition to questions of pleasure and modesty, privacy in the visiting room represents an opportunity for prisoners to rediscover themselves. In contrast, controlling privacy is an instrument of power. Charles, an inmate at Val-de-Reuil, doesn't hesitate to speak of "hints of the Inquisition on the part of the prison administration".

To be seen or not to be seen is an obsessive thought in detention. Nanou, an inmate at Bapaume, explains the frustrating power of surveillance: "Sometimes I want it so much, but as soon as I see a guard, I'm blocked. I'm very fearful, and every time I want to make love, it's the low wall that stops me." Over the years, paranoid reflexes have gradually inspired the "living together" reflexes taught in detention. The aim is to track down those who see, see those who know and recognize them, in keeping with the maxim that identifying one's enemies gives one a head start in all defense mechanisms. Prisoners are all the more aware of what surveillance represents, as they practice it among themselves and against the warders themselves. In prison, everyone is watching each other, and the only respite from this incessant vigil is to be found in the darkness of a cell, between each opening of the eyepiece signifying the surveillance rounds. This suffering is also expressed when prisoners make the certainty of not being seen their first requirement for conjugal encounters in prison.

Increasingly, both inside and out, the capacity for surveillance is being replaced and even amplified by the development of the *virtual eye* constituted by internal video circuits. The reflex of many inmates concerning the possibility of intimate visits leads them to insist that there should be no cameras filming their lovemaking. This fear, so often evoked, expresses the extent to which the feeling of being watched is omnipresent in prison. Any notion of *trust* and *intimacy* is associated with a form of *naivety*. Wardens are *hacks*, and *hacks* are civil servants paid to *watch*[235]. Looking at what others don't want to show is experienced by inmates as a form of punishment. This punishment is experienced as a dispossession of privacy, in a random situation, at the mercy of an actual gaze or not. There is humiliation in being seen, but also in the feeling of submission to the authority of the prison administration, which alternately holds the power to see or not to see. This question of intimacy stolen by surveillance is at the heart of prisoners' sexual preoccupations. Between a sexuality encouraged and aroused by the distribution of pornography, and the prohibition of sexual relations, between the fact that prisoners can be *watched at any time* in their sexual intimacy, including solitary, and the fact that masturbation is organized as an outlet for the deprivation of sexual relations, prison remains a place where the guilty must feel guilty.

---

235. The word *maton* first appeared in 1926 (Esnault), to designate a snitch. Then in 1946, again by the same author, *maton was* used to designate a guard. *Maton* comes from *mater*, "to observe", a word from Algiers French, and from *matar*, "to kill" (*Dictionnaire étymologique et historique du français*, Paris, Larousse/Bordas, 1998).

236

In flagrante delicto or the regression of guilt

In addition to the material impossibility of meeting a spouse during confinement, the loss of intimacy, coupled with the nagging and uncertain fear of being seen, is one of the main causes cited to describe sexual disturbances in detention. Bruno, an inmate at Val-de-Reuil, describes his troubles as follows: "I have erection problems that I didn't have before. I'm always afraid of being caught in the act. What disturbs my sexuality the most is the fear of being caught."

This fear of being "over-caught", described as the apprehension of being reproached for a fault, is also reminiscent of the refusal to be *caught*, in what sodomy represents of humiliation and submission. In prison, because sexual practices are hunted down, they belong to the shameful realm of a hidden exception, the better to escape the humiliation of disciplinary punishment. This is the regressive dimension of pleasure control that Daniel Gonin details when he concludes: "The administration feels itself to be the ambiguous guardian of this morality of displeasure. [...] Sex, on which the difference between beings is established, opens up a space for speech. This space, forbidden to the prisoner, plunges him back into indifferentiation."[236] This continual distrust of being seen or caught in flagrante delicto plunges inmates into a regressive relationship, and places supervisors in a parental role. The deprivation of freedom of movement is accepted as the basis of incarceration. On the other hand, any other dispossession is seen as an injustice, an abuse of power by an institution disguising its domination behind punitive accessories and security arguments. In this way, prison loses in respect what it gains in authority. This lends credence to Norbert Elias's assertion that "there is violence in society against institutions that do not keep their promises".

---

236. GONIN (Daniel), *op. cit.* p. 189.

Surrendering intimacy to the guards' *power of sight* places inmates in situations of continual avoidance to escape the stalking gaze. Talking about homosexual relations in the shadow of the cells, Damien, an inmate at Val-de-Reuil, explains: "It's very difficult, the mere sound of keys and footsteps, and the stress becomes paralyzing. Wanting to fuck in prison makes you go crazy." This is the sense in which the power to punish has evolved over the centuries, as Patricia O'Brien notes: "Prison not only aggravated physical weakness, it also caused a loss of identity and self-respect in the prisoner. [...] The new punishment was synonymous with sexual repression, isolation, estrangement, humiliation and could result in madness, depression or suicide."[237]

The "need for punishment" that each individual develops through the "feeling of guilt" referred to by Freud, is taken over by the institution, in place of the superego[238]. This represents an intrusion by the prison administration into the psychic intimacy of inmates, who as adults receive prescriptive injunctions of right and wrong from outside. The regressive phenomena provoked by imprisonment generate an exogenous guilt specific to the learning process, which erodes the existential autonomy of the individuals whom the institution promises to reintegrate, by replacing the endogenous control of desires, specific to adult life. This is social repression, where the same individuals are expected to function according to the repressive principles of individual morality. Beyond sexual questions understood as coital practice or the search for orgasm, the whole libidinal construction is subject to the authority of an administration that controls, distributes pornography, prohibits behavior, organizes the circumstances of encounters and condemns excesses. Undoubtedly, the totalizing aspects of prison find a particularly favorable outlet in questions of sexuality.

------

237. O'Brien (Patricia), *op. cit.* p. 54.
238. On how guilt functions as a control over desires, see Rabouin (David), *op. cit.* p. 112.

Bodily intimacy put to the test by searches

> "The strip search can be analyzed as a mortification rite imposed by the penitentiary institution. [...] For those subjected to it, it leads to a degradation of self-image and a desecration of identity."[239]

Encounters in the visiting room constitute a breach in the permeability between inside and outside. These moments of encounter justify the power of surveillance, which interferes with the intimacy of the body, the exhibition of sex and all material expressions of desire. In prison, this is the price of the encounter with otherness[240].

In the process of guarding, and in order to maintain authority over the mass of men guarded, the prison administration, in an unfavorable numerical relationship with respect to inmates, must base its disciplinary authority on its *ability to know*, to be aware of and to keep abreast of any breach or attempt at disobedience. This is the basis of surveillance, which consists of seeing and investigating, with complete disregard for privacy, in order to establish a permanent watertight seal. Ford, a prisoner at Œrmingen, recounts the discomfort of post-parlor searches: "I used to see my girlfriend every three weeks. But then I couldn't even go straight back to the visiting room for the search, because I had too much of a hard-on." The denial of privacy is so blatant that both accounts and analyses frequently equate strip-searching with rape. Respect for security conditions justifies the *"nothing in, nothing out"* rule. The principle of incarceration is based on the development of a confined existence, devoid of all outside attributes. By deduction, sexual relations symbolizing a fusion between inside and outside are rendered impossible.

---

239. GOFFMAN (Erving), *op. cit.* p. 64.
240. "Inmates must be searched frequently and as often as the head of the establishment deems necessary." Article D. 275 paragraph 1 of the New Code of Criminal Procedure.

The desire to know affects not only the body, but also every detail of the inmate's existence. The individual cell, understood as the spatial embodiment of each person's intimacy, is randomly scrutinized and analyzed. Objects are touched, moved, controlled, looked at, and the inmates can't ignore the way they maintain their libido, when they keep pornographic material, sexual accessories or even erotic letters. This is how Bruno, an inmate at Val-de-Reuil, describes the experience and consequences of searches of his individual cell: "We've made dildos out of cardboard, rags and condoms, and I've also got some gay DVDs. But when there's a search in the cell, the warders notice and they treat me badly." What each person is able to hide in the outside world in terms of sexual excitement and personal fantasies, all these objects as diverse as they are varied, likely to testify to the intimacy of practices, adventures or feelings, which only find their possible realization because they are kept secret, are exposed to a forced otherness in prison. Detention sifts through the whole of a prisoner's existence, from the smallest object to the tiniest desire, and the only way not to feel violated by the visit to the *home* that each prisoner reconstitutes for himself is to possess nothing, and to be content with the immaterialized possessions in his thoughts.

Whether it concerns men or women, strip-searching[241], as a violation of intimacy, is a humiliation, a violence suffered daily. It is no doubt illusory to overlook the fact that society at large will one day suffer the repercussions of this trampled dignity. The European Commissioner for Human Rights, Álvaro Gil-Robles, points out: "Under these conditions, people come out of there worse than they went in, full of hatred against the society that treated them this way." This opinion is observed today at all levels by those involved in incarceration, as this prison director

---

241. On the legal conditions governing searches, see HERZOG-EVANS (Martine), *La Gestion du comportement du détenu*, Paris, L'Harmattan, coll. "Logiques juridiques", 1998, pp. 160-164.

testifies: "It's obvious that detention fosters regression, humiliation and guilt, like body searches for example. It's the problem of the mule who brings home the bacon and is put under pressure. Grandparents have been caught with a hundred grams of pot, which they were supposed to bring to their grandson's visiting room. The women's pain doesn't spare them either, as their privacy is violated and their femininity disregarded: "You don't have time to undress before they've already said 'your panties', even when you're menstruating... It's humiliating enough as it is."[242]

However unpleasant they may be, these moments are justified by security conditions, the definition of which varies according to the wishes of authority as much as the many illegal practices that prisoners develop to escape disciplinary obedience[243]. And yet, the smell of cannabis is sufficiently pervasive in detention for its use to be more than just presumed: everyone knows that detention is amply stocked with illegal psychotropic substances, whose consumption the prison administration is suspected of tacitly supporting, to maintain a pseudo-serenity in the cells. To get around the *"I know but I don't know" rule*, trafficking is organized through natural orifices. As in the case of the ban on sexual relations in the visiting room, punishment is meted out at random, with a skilful balance between the desire to signify prohibition and authority on the one hand, and measured laxity on the other. Myriam, an inmate at Bapaume, describes her supply as follows: "I put my personal drink in my vagina, but I don't tamper with anything. We're strip-searched every time, but we don't go to the gynecologist! Except in Rennes, they did an ultrasound on me, and with what I was carrying, I got thirty days in the disciplinary ward."

---

242. Géraldine, 20, disadvantaged background, homicide, ten years old, for two and a half years, testimony *in* Rostaing (Corinne), *op. cit.*, p. 257.
243. See Veil (Claude) and Lhuilier (Dominique), (ed.), *op. cit.*, pp. 146-147.

Strip searches, in which inmates have to bend over and cough to get a clear view of the inside of their orifices, are therefore largely illusory in terms of effectiveness. Everyone knows this, yet no one does without it. It's as if this obligatory passage at the end of the visiting room were a security vestige whose sole purpose today is to remind inmates that the temporary rehabilitation of the *feeling of freedom* they may have experienced in the visiting room was only temporary. The strip search represents a second decompression chamber, through which inmates are reminded of the concept of submission, as a preamble to their return to detention. Armand, an inmate at Val-de-Reuil, waxes philosophical about this ritual moment, which reminds him of the army: "At the strip search, you have to cough, lower your ass... And even me, at 66, I have to comply with this practice! If you don't accept promiscuity, you're lost, it's part of the atmosphere."

Prison cannot deny what allows it to exist: it is an institution of legal exception. So, beyond the question of privacy in the visiting room, the very principle of confinement leads to a disappropriation of the self, to the benefit of an arbitrary appropriation of individuals by the prison administration. This is how Simone Buffard described this mechanism: "The search is not and cannot be a simple control operation; it affects the real body, the imaginary body and the symbolic body at the same time; the man searched is a man possessed."[244] Challenging the existence of such practices calls into question the very principle of authoritarian guarding. However, the intrusion of human rights and dignity into security issues calls for a "joint philosophical revision of the two dimensions of security - external and internal security - which can be the lever for real change"[245]. Technical developments suggest that the humiliation of strip-searching could be replaced by electronic detectors

---

244. Buffard (Simone), *op. cit.* p. 47.
245. Veil (Claude) and Lhuilier (Dominique), (ed.), *op. cit.*, p. 156.

or visualization methods, the physiological harmlessness of which has yet to be demonstrated.

It's also the harshness of this exposure that underpins the demand for intimate visits. Prisoners' avowed intentions lie not so much in the desire to practice sexuality, as in a desire to survive, to experience moments away from the obsessive gaze of the prison administration, privileged moments that no one would witness. It's a search for *parcels of reality*, as opposed to the artificial survival of a guarded existence within walls. Because prison steals everything and dispossesses people, each person wants to reconstitute a *patch of* intimacy, inaccessible from the point of view of the prison authorities.

The conjugal dimension in the shadow of walls

> "We must never underestimate the fact that most people love, love to be loved, need to be lovable, to have relatively peaceful relationships. Being able to be kind to others goes a long way towards defusing violence."[246]

Irrespective of the concerns of prisoners themselves, confinement generously produces significant consequences for their spouses. Isolation not only deprives the convicted person of emotional and sexual ties. Very often, imprisonment is a couple affair. To speak only of prisoners is to omit, for many of them, the part of themselves that represents them on the outside. In this sense, punishing prisoners is also punishing their spouses. In view of the importance attributed to the couple and the family entity, from a political, legal and social point of view, the deprivation imposed by prison underlines the scale of the price that

---

246. ENRIQUEZ (Eugène) and HAROCHE (Claudine), *La Face obscure des démocraties modernes*, Érès, coll. "Sociologie clinique", Ramonville Saint-Agne, 2002, p. 96.

society intends to make people pay for disorders caused to property, people or institutions. Even if this deprivation is not an objective, we cannot deny that it is used as an instrument to assert the power of guardianship, and thus to make the punitive institution even more dissuasive. As far as maintaining family ties is concerned, this situation contradicts the official objectives stated and expressed as pious hopes by politicians[247]: "The prisoner's family must not be treated as if it were equally responsible for the offence committed, as was the case under the Ancien Régime justice system [...] maintaining family ties is essential for the future reintegration of convicts"[248]

While all the findings suggest that the resocialization of individuals cannot do without the two essential elements of work and housing on release, the fact remains that the best bulwark against recidivism is to maintain the emotional environment of family and friends, seen as the essential reception environment to prevent ex-offenders from returning to risky frames of reference. This is how inmates view their release with optimism. The couple and the family represent points of reference that enable them to escape from the totalizing world of prison, and to remember that confinement is an exception when liberation is the goal. In this perspective, sexuality, associated with seduction and the certainty of existing as an object of desire for others, is described as the antidote to self-loathing. Fabrice, incarcerated in Val-de-Reuil, talks about the support he expects from his wife's affection, after hating himself for the sexual offence he committed: "The tender relationship as a couple in

---

247. In the same vein, see the report of the European Committee for the Prevention of Torture and Inhuman or Degrading Treatment or Punishment (CPT): *Report to the Government of the French Republic by the CPT*, article 133, Brussels, January 19 1993.
248. Assemblée nationale, Mermaz (Louis), (président, Floch (Jacques), (rapporteur), Commission d'enquête sur la situation dans les prisons françaises, "La France face à ses prisons", rapport n° 2521, Paris, 2000, tome I (rapport, 328 pages) and tome II (auditions, 565 pages).

the visiting room, and everything we can do there, for me it's essential to reassure myself about my self-confidence, and about the contrast between who I am now compared to who I was before my offence."

A couple's survival of the prison break

Long-sentence confinement creates surreal expectations for couples. In addition to temporal conditions, the regression felt by inmates in their compulsion to obey the prison administration is also felt by their spouses, who have to submit to searches, shamelessness, frustration and the risk of having their visiting rights revoked if sexual behavior is observed. The authority of the administration is representative of the father who decides and punishes. When the inmates become accustomed to this notion of authority and obedience, which they endure in the day-to-day life of detention, the spouses suffer this regressive situation, like collateral damage not taken care of by society.

Through the break-up it causes over time, prison deprives conjugal relationships of the sensory and carnal bond represented by sexuality. The consequences are the "evils" that Étienne Dumont described in 1818, assuming that only men were victims[249]. The survival of couples must be motivated by a rewriting of the relationship with the other, in which the carnal aspect is lacking[250]. Many *long-suffering prisoners* are left by their partners, for whom waiting outside the walls eliminates any prospects. Moreover, the circumstances of the separation give greater scope for infidelity, and although few inmates express this concern, many choose to break up at the start of a long sentence. They argue that

---

249. On the prejudices linked to the impossible union of bodies, see DUMONT (Étienne), *Théorie des peines et des récompenses*, Paris/Londres, Bossange et Masson, 1818, tome I, p. 388.
250. MONTANDON (Cléopâtre) and CUETTAZ (Bernard), *Paroles de gardiens, paroles de détenus. Bruits et silences de l'enfermement*, Genève, Masson, coll. "Déviance et société", 1981, p. 141.

"imprisonment is more painful for two", and by breaking up, they find a way out of a relationship understood as an exclusive love and sexual relationship, made impossible by the separation of bodies. For some, it's easier to give up on a dream they no longer believe in, by anticipating a separation they suspect will be unbearable. So as not to add to the humiliation of condemnation and confinement, the equation that seems to prevail in incarceration is *rather leave than be left*. Some openly explain that they don't want to feel like the obvious, official "cuckold".

Finally, one of the justifications for breaking up is the delicacy of not imposing such a disturbing and incomplete relationship on a woman they don't want to victimize. Sexual abstinence or furtive practices in the visiting room are ultimately the best way to deal with couples who find themselves in circumstances too far removed from their usual points of reference. The sexuality stolen from visiting rooms is mechanical, hygienic, animal and devoid of seduction. The temptation to end the relationship then appears to be the solution best suited to incarceration. This, for example, is the choice made by Jason, an inmate at Saint-Mihiel: "At first, I was very impatient for visiting hours. After a while, it became routine, and I even ended up refusing out of respect for her. In the end, it's disgusting how sex happens here. I preferred to cut all ties so it wouldn't be so hard." This is also the point of view of Ford, detained at Œrmingen: "I took it out on her so that she ended up leaving me. I received her badly, telling her in every visiting room, 'I didn't ask you to come!' It hurt me that she was suffering because of me. And then here, spouses are badly received, and the wardens flirt with our girlfriends. They act proud because they're free."

Sexual relations involve two actors, a space and time. The conditions of the visiting room modify these three parameters. On the one hand, intimacy is not respected, as the closeness of some mingles with the closeness of others, in a spectacle that is as deviously concealed as it is collective. On the other hand, the space devoted to conjugal encounters doesn't lend itself to excitement, and from week to week, invariably boils down to two chairs and a table in a cubicle with half-height walls. Finally, the mastery of time to build excitement is neither the prerogative of lovers, nor at the service of excitement, since sexuality boils down to the timed challenge of *doing without being seen*.

Rumor has it that women at liberty remain more faithful to their imprisoned partners than their male counterparts, who are accused of being quick to console themselves after a separation. Experience also tells us that, when it comes to love, generalities are often shortcuts that do little to reflect realities that are as diverse as they are varied. Prison frequently represents the occasion of a marital break-up, of which inmates are invariably the actors or the victims. This bitter and worrying observation is common to all studies on prison. The deprivation of conjugal sexual relations is analyzed as a destabilizing factor for couples, due to the disruption of self-image and the estrangement caused by confinement. This is also Corinne Rostaing's observation: "This absence of relations affects the individual in his personal life, making the man doubt his virility and the woman her femininity. [...] The denial of sexuality explains the difficulties, even the failure, of certain marital relationships. Imbalance within the couple is at the root of many suicides."[251]

During the interviews, the men seemed particularly respectful of the freedom their wives enjoy outside the home, and therefore recognize women's sexuality as a need similar to that of men. Of course, it's hard to say whether these responses are tinged with reassuring illusions, or whether the inmates preferred not to verbalize the possibility of being

---

251. ROSTAING (Corinne), *op. cit.*, p. 132.

cheated on, to safeguard their self-esteem. It's always easier to be a *lord* when the balance of power isn't in your favor. Prisoners are aware that they are in a position of weakness, due to the material and emotional dependence they feel on the outside world. For some of them, women, in their role as indispensable helpers, are likened to mothers whose feelings cannot be questioned. This is the case, for example, of Geronimo, a prisoner in Val-de-Reuil, who met his partner in prison and is now married to the mother of one of his friends, with whom, of course, he has never shared a sexual relationship: "She helps me rebuild myself. [...] If she were unfaithful, I wouldn't hold it against her. I'm tolerant."

Tenderness and love or the metaphors of sexual need
"The measure of love is to love without measure"[252]

Because in everyone's mind, sexuality is frequently linked to the notion of the couple and the global parameters that underpin it, the influences of the prohibition of sexual relations are interdependent with sentimental frustrations, as Irène Théry's analyses show when she defines the couple as "a story and a conversation"[253]. Carnal closeness is not necessarily understood as the search for orgasmic pleasure. For many inmates, they are above all an expression of feelings, evoked from the angle of a reassuring tenderness. To exist for someone is what is at stake in the encounter with otherness that the visiting room offers. These are also the limits of what discipline allows. In prison, otherness is only accessible at a distance that obeys a limit virtualized by discipline.

---

252. This quote is attributed to St. Augustine, from a sermon in which he states more precisely, "The measure of loving God is God himself; the measure of this love is to love him without measure."
253. Théry (Irène), "La côte d'Adam. Retour sur le paradoxe démocratique", *Esprit*, no 273, March-April 2001.

The fusional relationship that Plato describes when he explains that everyone is inclined to find their other half[254] corresponds to the desire for fusion that inmates evoke in their search for tenderness. Such an encounter is reassuring for everyone, and particularly for those in whom Freud identifies a "libido turned towards love life"[255]. When prison provokes regressions to childhood, existential anxieties find salvation in expressions of affection reminiscent of the satisfactions of a loving, reassuring mother. Prisons are reminiscent of childhood, when they act as punishing ascendants. Moreover, it is not the offence committed that is the main basis for guilt. From the point of view of potential victims, it's much more the guilt of having been caught at fault.

Among the words used to describe the suffering of incarceration, *family* and *friendship* invariably come to mind. Lack of tenderness is described as never being in contact with the body of a fellow human being. This does not necessarily imply sexuality in the genital sense. Tom, a prisoner at Œrmingen, explains the disturbances in his sexuality: "It's because I'm missing the essential. That is, a woman next to me, not just for sex, but also for love and tenderness. In fact, for me, sex has never been possible without love. For the inmates, it's a question of remembering their condition as living beings by confronting the humanity of the other through a physical exchange. Prisoners seek to escape the loneliness of daily life through the reality of sleeping alone. Armand confides: "When I go to bed in the evening, I get close to my duffel bag, but it's not my wife. It's hard to get into a cold bed and sleep alone."[256]

Except in the case of prisoners with a particularly high libido, sexuality in the sense of the search for orgasm is rarely identified as the main

---

254. PLATO, *op. cit.* p. 115.
255. FREUD (Sigmund), *Des types libidinaux, op. cit.*, pp. 5-6.
256. Armand is 66 years old. He is incarcerated at the Val-de-Reuil detention center.

lack. On the other hand, the collateral aspects of sexuality, through the management of emotional relationships with spouses or family, are defined as the hardest thing to live[257] in incarceration. In fact, it's often identified as the only truly disturbing thing, a disturbance for which there is no palliative. Hippocampe, an inmate at Val-de-Reuil, confides: "It's simply the lack of affection, the lack of female presence and human warmth in general that is lacking night and day."

For the prison administration, the tenderness in question quickly becomes a source of disorder and shamelessness, as soon as it involves touching a body. And yet, in their discourse, prison guards seem to tolerate physical contact as long as it doesn't involve the genitals or areas of the body commonly recognized as erogenous. Generally speaking, incarceration creates a dichotomy between sustained and growing desires, an unfulfilled need for tenderness, and an arousal often exacerbated by an overconsumption of virtual sexual objects: "I've come to hate my sex so much I don't like masturbating. I'm never satisfied. [...] I've often thought of cutting off my penis. [...] The lack of affection, the lack of tenderness that comes from caressing, from the sexual act, has made me aggressive, nasty and dangerous."[258]

This situation is not without creating disorder in the lives of *long-sentenced prisoners,* who, on release, will have to compensate for shortcomings while balancing their desires in their encounter with an otherness that has not suffered the same damage, as E. Swinnen explains: "Many ex-prisoners say it clearly: they are no longer capable of loving. They go

---

257. GRAVIER (Bruno) and LAMOTHE (Pierre), "La sexualité en prison: un comportement à risque?", paper presented at the 5th International AIDS Conference, Montreal, June 4-9, 1989, p. 166.
258. Raymond R., detained at Saint-Martin-de-Ré for sixteen years *in* MONNEREAU (Alain), *op. cit.* p. 107.

through life with a kind of indifference from which they cannot free themselves."[259]

Censorship of carnal encounters thwarts nagging desires. The loneliness of incarceration is a daily occurrence, and nothing short of over-activity or numbing with legal or illegal psychotropic drugs can overcome the sense of isolation of *long sentences*. The tenderness and voluptuousness of sexual pleasure are described as the most effective antidotes to the rigors of prison, understood as an institution as dehumanized as it is dehumanizing, in which human relationships are vitiated by violence and self-interest. Prison is synonymous with darkness, as opposed to women themselves, synonymous with tenderness and affection. Prison often boils down to a sum of individual solitudes forming a constrained collective. According to Armand, an inmate at Val-de-Reuil, the emotional misery of some inmates sometimes translates into the need to telephone to hear a voice whisper something in the privacy of an ear, in the illusion of a privileged relationship: "Most here have no one left in their lives. Some call 12 or the talking clock to hear someone speak to them and feel like they're making a phone call!"

Creating new couples

The months leading up to release are often spent looking for a new partner, to ensure the transition between inside and outside. Yet prison is experienced as a circumstance that leaves its indelible mark on every episode of life. So, often, the purity of sentimental demands cannot be envisaged within the walls. Charles testifies: "We waited for a parole to really get together. The important thing was to make sure it didn't happen in prison." For other inmates, isolation seems insurmountable.

---

259. SWINNEN (E.), *op. cit.* p. 280.

Once in prison, the process of recruiting a partner begins[260]. The sexual dimension is very present in this quest, which also serves to create the illusion of exclusive possession of an object of excitement, while reassuring oneself by becoming someone's other.

Contingencies and objectives

The new relationships forged from within are utilitarian, responding on both sides to a desire that is not necessarily sentimental. Prisoners recruit women as they would recruit an object, with no prior respect for a physical or epistolary encounter. Augustin, an inmate at Saint-Mihiel, has witnessed the practices of his fellow inmates: "They give each other addresses, girlfriends they know, sluts whose addresses they have. It's a form of solidarity. [...] Generally speaking, sluts are frequent at discos and less frequent on the street...".

The market for couples between inside and outside, obeys well-thought-out interests between the protagonists. Male inmates are very much in demand for psychological support for some, and sexuality for others. In both cases, it's a question of existing for someone of the opposite sex, in a relationship of complicity that contrasts with the paranoia organized by detention. It's also about orchestrating a symbolic escape from the self, by building an intimacy outside the bars, through which the partner spouse makes a part of the self exist in society outside. Some seek a woman who will take on the traits of a loving, comforting mother. Others will seek to express fantasies and represent an object

---

260. As a reminder, in 2009, even though the prison population is allowed to own a computer, internet connections are impossible and forbidden. To organize meetings between partners, the only option is to use classified ads in magazines. In addition, the possession of cell phones is forbidden, even though the number of mobiles circulating in prison is particularly high. In keeping with the principle of watertightness that governs confinement, and with varying degrees of success, the institution strives to control access to the outside world, even if this access is immaterial.

of excitement for their partner. In all cases, the aim is to reconstitute the symbolic or real otherness that imprisonment eliminates through monosexual confinement.

Women's interests in responding to such solicitations are varied. In some cases, the thirst for sexuality combined with the loneliness of some, sometimes responds to the desire for immigration of others. In other words, the material and emotional destitution of some women on the outside echoes the loneliness of men on the inside. Jason, an inmate at Saint-Mihiel, observes this phenomenon, and deduces: "Often it's the women who advertise. Some women want men with a mean streak. Others want protection. It's all *calculated, it's not really a meeting*." Similarly, the emotional destitution of prisoners is exploited by women looking for a sham marriage to come and stay in France. There's a market in the classified ads, where male prisoners looking for a wife are willing to pay for a foreign woman to travel and settle in temporarily, agreeing to marry a French prisoner whose photo she knows only, in order to establish herself in France. Karim, a prisoner in Val-de-Reuil, explains how these falsely fortuitous unions work: "They correspond *via* magazines like *Itinérant* or *Anima*, a magazine for black women. They're in Africa. They write and then it's 'I love you' right away, then 'I don't have any money', so they send for them. They have to deprive themselves of everything, so they come, get married here in prison and they stay in France."

This market seems so accessible that some of the inmates we met suspect the existence of a network, organized by "pimps from outside" who would allow foreign women to come to France in return for a fee, often paid by the inmate's family. On both sides, these unspoken contracts are a response to situations of distress, akin to survival issues, between men and women in extreme situations. Officially, these marriages are not consummated, insofar as nothing is stipulated in the facilities' internal regulations.

The future lovers correspond by mail, sending photos of each other. Then comes the telephone phase, which allows them to identify a voice and thus embody a sensuality. Finally, these women begin the administrative process of obtaining access to the visiting room, and their bodies exalt, to the extent of the disciplinary risk, these desires too long contained by confinement. The respective needs of male and female prisoners are instrumentalized in the form of a more or less official union, the purpose of which is to correct the frustrations caused by confinement, but also the wounds of previous existence on the outside. There is nothing to suggest that these couples will survive after release. The team of psychologists at Val-de-Reuil notes that couples formed in this way in prison generally do not survive the changeover on release. Yet the idea of leaving a long sentence in the company of someone with whom everything will once again be possible is a reassuring one.

These new couples represent a challenge to the walls of the prison, which these women and men bypass. Nanou, an inmate at Bapaume, describes the excitement of her new relationship, which contrasts with the violence she experienced before: "It was fate that brought us together. It was love at first sight at the prison. As fate would have it, we'd already been in love thirty years before. I had no family and nobody came to see me. I would have killed myself. He's tender, cuddly, smiling. He has a large fortune. Out there with him, I'm guaranteed happiness."

Detention centers where men and women are housed in separate, perfectly impermeable units, give rise to other types of play. At Bapaume, the exercise yard has a dividing wall between the men's and women's units. It's from here that encounters begin, culminating in frequent unions within the same prison. Men and women talk to each other behind the wall, without ever meeting visually. The second phase consists of an exchange of love bills, followed by letters in which the inmates include a photo. These restrictive meeting conditions, known as *"parloirs sauvages"*, are accepted as the only palliative to existential loneliness. As Béa, an inmate at Bapaume, explains: "You talk to the first person, then the second, and if you're not interested, you give up and pass on the details to someone else. This relationship represents a rebirth that she views with optimism, and for her represents the only possible tomorrow: "I was in a cocoon, life for me stopped. I died in prison, but with him, I'll rise again."

The sexual aura of the kingpin

In contrast to the sense of degradation and *devirilization of* the prisoner's condition due to the constraints of confinement, many male prisoners represent a sexual symbol of virility and power on the outside. The myth of the prisoner *thirsty for sex* because of a lack of women, is frequently associated with the myth of the delinquent whose virility is underlined by his capacity to disobey order, his insubordination and his resistance to authority. All parameters that suggest a sexual potency equivalent to the history that precedes them, to finally outline the contours of the *most exciting man*. As a result, prison mailrooms are inundated with letters from women expressing their desire for a particularly high-profile inmate, whose adventures give him an undeniable aura. Today's kingpins continue to hold a fascination for women. This aura attests to the reversal of presumed values implicit in the Manichean vision of the prison institution. Prisoners represent evil through the offence they have committed, and at the same time enjoy a reputation for seductiveness and virility. The warders represent goodness through the corrective function they perform, and at the same time enjoy a dubious appreciation on the part of women, who judge their function pejoratively. Where bandits are heroes, wardens are obedient, submissive, emasculated anti-heroes, at the service of an institution that protects them. Their virility is nothing in itself; it requires the support of a superior authority who directs them and a set of rules that endorse them.

This mythologized image of the two social groups is not general, but in the last resort, men know that only women will be the judges of this reality, and that their libidinal power will depend on this opinion. This aura is not without influence on behavior between men in detention; in fact, some inmates complain that wardens try to seduce their wives when they enter or leave the visiting rooms. Because they have power over inmates based on the freedom they possess and the hierarchy that justifies their position, supervisors exercise their prerogatives of seduction in the very places where inmates cannot. These behaviors attest to the fact that men compete with each other by evaluating their power to seduce.

Chapter 3
Outlook

"[...] any innocent amusement that human art can invent is useful from a double point of view: 1o for the pleasure itself that results from it; 2o by its tendency to weaken those dangerous inclinations that man has by nature. And when I speak of innocent amusements, I mean all those that cannot be shown to be harmful. Their introduction being conducive to the happiness of society, it is the duty of the legislator to encourage them, or at least not to hinder them."[261]

Today, more than ever before, the debate on sexual freedom penetrates the prison sphere. The influences of experiments carried out in foreign countries over the last few decades are realities that are hard to ignore. By dint of criticizing prison for its criminogenic effects and its notorious inability to reintegrate de-socialized individuals, the concept of incarceration is entering a new phase of reform. Either we accept the counter-productive effects of an institution "which cannot be dispensed with"[262], and we instrumentalize the confinement of a specific category of the population, in exponential proportions; this is the American model which is gradually leading to the industrialization of the punitive

---

261. BENTHAM (Jeremy), *op. cit.* p. 244.
262. FOUCAULT (Michel), *op. cit.* p. 234.

system analyzed by Nils Christie[263], culminating in the contemporary phenomenon of the stock market listing of private prison companies. In other words, the many disadvantages resulting from the disruption caused by the prison institution confirm the contradiction between the ambitions of a relative order of society, in which freedom for all is a general principle, and deprivation an exception. This conception is the theoretical contribution of the reformers, and it is in this direction that the recent desire to introduce the opportunity for conjugal encounters is timidly taking shape. Prisoners and their families are the direct beneficiaries of this development. In view of the satisfaction of this process, it is society as a whole, and the restoration of a social bond, that is the secondary beneficiary of this new prerogative. In practice, the legislator conceives this process with the aim of obtaining added value while maintaining the essential attributes of the power to punish.

Prisoners' expectations and reservations

The deprivation of sexual relations is generally accepted as an integral part of the *quantum of* the prison sentence. Despite the suffering caused by the deprivation of carnal encounters, despite the lack of otherness from both an emotional and a sexual point of view, each and every inmate remains skeptical about the proposed changes to the visiting rooms, of which the prison administration does not keep them informed. The daily grind of sentencing, the psychotropic drugs consumed and the difficulty of a general rebellion, have overcome any hint of official change in the area of conjugal encounters, apart from a gradual shift in the *cursor of authority*, increasingly expressed in the form of a more flexible interpretation of the principle of prohibiting sexual relations in the visiting room. Prison militancy has only two faces: mutiny or

---

263. *Christie* (Nils), *L'Industrie de la punition. Prison and penal policy in the West*, Paris, Autrement, 2003, p. 19.

gradual individual disobedience, aimed at gradually and implicitly gaining prerogatives that only the law can ratify[264].

Reconstructing the outside

Prisoners have a clear vision of what they expect from an evolution in their right to privacy. They also have a few fears, which they base in particular on an already tainted relationship of trust with the prison administration, as evidenced by Stewart's naive question: "And would there or wouldn't there be cameras in the bungalows?"

The constraint of being seen is so omnipresent in the workings of the prison, that the idea of a system that does not involve surveillance seems as implausible as it is inaccessible. What's more, a sexuality suddenly made possible cannot be imagined without a few reservations, analyzed here as an *a priori* mistrust of a new prerogative that would conceal its discomforts. Myriam, a female prisoner we met in Bapaume, benefited from the experimentation of Family Visiting Units (UVF) when she was incarcerated at the women's prison in Rennes. She experienced her first meeting not without a few misgivings. Finding herself face-to-face with her fiancé in the peaceful setting of the recently opened UVF, while remaining aware that she was still within the prison walls, seemed surreal at first: "It felt strange to see him so close to me, I didn't really believe it. It was strange to know that he was in prison with me too. At first, I thought we were being watched all the time. [...] In fact, it was a good memory, it went well after a few hours, and eventually, I ended up forgetting that I was in prison."

---

264. Prisoners do not have the right of association enjoyed by free individuals in the outside world, even for cultural purposes. This rule is customary. The Conseil d'Etat has ruled on the right of assembly, considering that detainees "cannot usefully avail themselves of the provisions of the laws of June 30, 1881 and March 28, 1907 relating to freedom of assembly". CE, ref., May 27 2005, *Observatoire international des prisons*, no 280866 (AJDA 2005, p. 1579).

This reappropriation of the ability to live without the authority of the gaze of those who have the power to punish, is seen as an essential phase for *long sentences to* recover a measure of autonomy before returning to life on the outside. This concept, which has long been shared across the Atlantic (notably in Canada), is now being championed by the Ministry of Justice, which has drawn on the conclusions of the three phases of UVF experimentation to decide to extend the process[265]. This project bears witness to a gradual recognition of the damaging effects of incarceration for *long sentences*, due to a double rupture: the first caused by incarceration, the second by release.

UVF is not seen as a measure of clemency. Rather, they are perceived as a development that is ultimately constrained by European recommendations, which are becoming harder to ignore with each passing year. It's a question of temporarily suspending the execution of the sentence, by staging a meeting within the prison walls, in the heart of a setting that represents the reality on the outside.

Prisoners want to forget the conditions of their incarceration, by "recovering" a sense of intimacy sheltered from surveillance and disciplinary sanctions. This gamble is only possible with the complicity of both the prison administration and the inmate population, according to respective commitments that position each in a quasi-contractual adult-to-adult context. The scheme is designed to provide an opportunity to reclaim autonomy, while temporarily erasing the feeling of submission to the punitive system.

---

265. In 2006, the prison administration made public its intention to extend the installation of UVFs following the conclusions of the experiments decided by the previous government and carried out at the Rennes women's detention center, and at the Poissy and Saint-Martin-de-Ré detention centers.

The spatio-temporal conditions of the encounter

"A small studio reproducing living conditions on the outside" is the recurring wish of the inmates we interviewed. Behind this statement lies the desire to forget the conditions of confinement, the dilapidation or precarious comfort of detention, and to ensure that the prison administration will have no possible regard for conjugal reunions. The space is described as having to be "human and welcoming", as opposed to the rigorous security of prison architecture.

Before any mention of sleeping, the inmates unanimously ask for a table and chairs, as if to express that the reunion that gives rise to seduction begins around a face-to-face discussion in a convivial spirit. The seated position is described as a socializing posture, allowing for more intimate encounters. These descriptions contrast with the more animalistic conception of a hygienic sexuality fueled by pornography in detention. The conjugal encounter is seen as an opportunity to rediscover the dignity of the outside world, embodied by a willing and, why not, loving partner. In contrast to the supine position of masturbation on a bed in front of the TV screen, the sexual encounter in the visiting room is intended to be the moment when the man stands up straight, physically, consciously and symbolically.

Sexuality and hygiene were closely linked in the interviews. The need for a watering hole was frequently mentioned. This underlines the importance of the body envelope - one's own and one's partner's - in the carnal encounter. *Cleanliness* is the key to uninhibited, uninhibited sexuality. It's as much a question of preparing the body before offering it to the other, as of erasing all traces of lovemaking on returning to prison. This modesty expresses the desire not to make visible the occurrence of practices that belong to the intimate, as opposed to today's visiting rooms, in which the intentions and practices of each person are deciphered as soon as they are dressed, on the arrival of visitors.

Depending on the aspirations of each individual, this *special parlor is intended to* be considered a *haven of peace, according to the* respective expectations of the inmates. While some aspire to tenderness, others expect sensuality, escape or comfort, as Armand's description testifies: "I would dream of a tea dance, with guests and more if affinities, in an atmosphere of seduction and pleasure, a convivial relationship, each with his feminine complement." According to the wishes heard, the marital meeting place should temporarily erase the sensations of confinement, giving the opportunity to reconstitute the cycle of a day's existence, with the satisfaction of going to bed and getting up in a state of weightlessness that recalls the outside while making us forget the inside. These reunions are nourished by an idyllic vision of the sensations outside, imagined over the years of confinement as an *El Dorado to be rediscovered*. The frequency of these meetings varies from once a week to twice a month. Weekends are considered the most opportune time for conjugal encounters. This almost dreamlike dimension of what could be the conditions for conjugal encounters in prison is thought up by the inmates, who nevertheless find it hard to believe in this new prerogative. It's worth noting that the conjugal encounters scheme is likened to an *old-fashioned* fantasy. While those of them who have already tasted this moment during previous incarcerations in other nations, prioritize their wish with less detail: "The place is secondary, the possibility of having it is paramount."[266]

The desire for a place with an ambiguous destination

Prisoners are very concerned that the layout of the facility should not represent a constraint to the practice of sexual relations. Behind this wish lie both issues of modesty, and concerns that the encounter with the partner could turn into a *sexual challenge*. Geronimo, an inmate at Val-de-Reuil, describes his wishes as follows: "Modesty needs to be

---

266. Wolf is 56 years old. He is a German national. We met him outside after he was released for health reasons.

reassured. We need to be able to have relations, but not necessarily sexual ones. It shouldn't be written on the door 'you're going to fuck!'"

The idea of assigning a place to the exclusive purpose of sexual practices is problematic for both warders and inmates, insofar as the former become accomplices to practices that the latter cannot hide. This is why, without carrying out a radical reform of the current visiting rooms, some inmates, including Bruno, would be happy with curtains between each cubicle, leaving each one free to experience the meeting in the visiting room in a platonic way, or, on the contrary, to develop a more intimate relationship: "It would be like a brothel, but the curtain wouldn't necessarily be closed."

Generally speaking, the expectations of prisoners are not very demanding. Their proposals are mostly realistic and sometimes even timid, inspired more by the sexual parlor system that exists in Hispanic countries, than by the development of a living space. The modesty of such a wish would make it easy, quick and inexpensive to implement. The first requirement is for them to escape the gaze of the guards and other visitors, and to be guaranteed a minimum of privacy, which today is largely denied in the prison environment. Dignity is considered both for themselves and for the partners who come to the visiting room. The two social groups represented in prison - the prison administration on the one hand, and the inmates on the other - refuse to let visiting rooms become "fuckodromes". While the wardens feel devalued by seeing their authority instrumentalized as a *guardian of modesty*, the inmates reject the idea that their spouses might be imagined to come to the visiting room as prostitutes. The stakes of this self-esteem lie as much in sincere respect for the women they love as in the self-image devalued by the obvious reminder of the animality of a purely sexual need. As Max, a prisoner at Œrmingen, explains: "We have to make sure that the warders don't say to themselves: 'She's here to get shot!'"

The demand for possible sexuality lies not so much in the possibility of practices, as in the conditions under which they take place. The opening of a place specifically dedicated to sexual practices is seen as an additional power given to the prison administration to regulate inmates' sex lives. In the same way that prison guards take prisoners to the shower, to training courses or to the infirmary, the idea that they should also take them to the den of conjugal sexuality is seen as a further intrusion into private life, more akin to added enslavement than regained dignity. The visiting room must remain a privileged moment that each person inhabits in his or her own way, with no supposed destination for the activities that take place there. Augustin explains: "I don't like premeditated acts. It reminds me of prostitution."[267]

Male inmates also fear that the designated specificity of a room dedicated to sexual relations will subject them to an *obligation of result* vis-à-vis their partner. They evoke the idea of a "challenge", forcing them to perform a sexual act that they don't necessarily feel they need to perform at the moment when the circumstances of the visiting room are dictated to them. As in life on the outside, they express the need to be in control of their libido in terms of quantity, occurrence and action. The possibility of an erectile failure[268] is half-expressed behind the apprehension of an exclusively sexual visiting room. With such premeditation in sexual occurrences, men fear they are no longer masters of their desires, and are instead subject to an external injunction to be aroused first, then perform.

Opinions on what could be a conjugal meeting place differ according to each person's sexual needs. If, generally speaking, the place should leave some doubt as to its main purpose, the inmates who

---

267. Augustin is 21 years old. He is incarcerated at the Saint-Mihiel detention center.
268. FALCONNET (Georges) and LEFAUCHEUR (Nadine), *op. cit.*, p. 92.

declare that they consume hygienic sexuality in the visiting room in its current configuration, or those whose sexual need is defined as vital and unsubstitutable, are already accustomed to the idea of uninhibited sexuality in all circumstances. For them, the fears of a spatio-temporal device implying the realization of an expected sexual performance are unfounded.

Improving the experience of confinement and its paradoxes

Without rejecting improvements in prison conditions, inmates are above all attached to the idea of minimizing the time spent incarcerated, with an undisguised impatience to get back to life, *the real life*, that of the outside world. The idea of seeing the prison regime reconstitute the conditions of the outside world within the walls, is closely associated with the fear of seeing these new measures replace the legal but unenforced prevalence of resocialization through the mechanisms of permissions[269] or parole[270]. In France, official figures show that the mechanisms used to release prisoners temporarily before their final release are used very sparingly: 82% of prisoners are released at the end of their sentence without ever having benefited from legal leave[271]. And yet, among the wishes expressed by the prison population in terms of conjugal relationships, is the desire to rediscover their bearings and tame their sexuality under the conditions of freedom. Beyond a furtive carnal rapprochement, the spatio-temporal opportunity for which is *ultimately* decided by the prison administration, the conjugal encounter is intended to represent a real escape from prison life. The voluptuousness of sex and tenderness hardly rhymes with the reality of a prison that *soils* everything it comes near. Organized sexuality within the prison

---

269. Article 723 of the Code of Criminal Procedure.
270. Articles 729 of the Code of Criminal Procedure.
271. International Prison Observatory, *Le Guide du prisonnier*, Paris, La Découverte, 2004, p. 447.

walls is seen both as a relief from the length of incarceration, and as an intrusion of the institution into the experience of intimacy.

From the opportunity for carnal closeness, many of the inmates interviewed expect the expression of the beauty of feelings and the quintessence of tenderness through the fusion of self with the chosen otherness. These emotions are contradicted by the prison world, which is described as dirty, repulsive, unfair and painful. For others, because everything that belongs to prison is stamped with an indelible and perverse memory, whatever the device, the walls will always represent a nightmarish environment that soils the ideals of love.

Behind these speeches lies a strong fear of ostracism, expressed as the fear of a population that recognizes itself as subject to a system. If everything becomes possible in prison, if the institution reproduces with too much precision the conditions outside, the recourse to confinement and the lengthening of sentences would become morally uncomplicated. The majority of the prison population represents the underprivileged rather than the *well-off*. Aware of this factor, prisoners do not want to constitute a social group that society would lock up at will, based on specifically defined illegalisms, in the manner of penal policy in the USA[272]. The organization of sexuality within the prison itself is also seen as an added submission to a system which, not satisfied with locking up a specific population, would also take on the task of organizing their existences, right down to the singularities of intimacy. The detainee population is not fooled by a punitive system

---

272. The incarceration rate in France is ninety-one inmates per one hundred thousand inhabitants, while the incarceration rate in the USA is seven hundred and fourteen inmates per one hundred thousand inhabitants [i.e. over 1% of the adult population in 2008, [*nda*], with a proportion of people of color exceeding 80% in some cities. WACQUANT (Loïc), "De l'État social à l'État carcéral. L'emprisonnement des 'classes dangereuses' aux États-Unis", *Le Monde diplomatique*, no. 532, July 1998.

that it considers to be unjustly instrumentalized for the benefit of a social order from which it does not benefit. This is Foucault's awareness of *popular illegalisms* justifying prison repression[273]. Even if they do not retract their guilt, inmates describe themselves as victims of a society in which they have not found their place, or in which their apprenticeship to life has been prevented by adults whose behavior goes unpunished. The idea that the prison administration prefers to organize their own sexuality within the walls, rather than benefiting from the furloughs or other conditional releases provided for by law, only reinforces the fear of seeing their existence dedicated to the prison institution, like an inescapable destiny, that of the ostracized and the recluse. UVF versus *conditional sentences:* a dreaded form of unfair competition. Some inmates have even evoked an illusory negotiation between accepting the ban on sexual relations, in exchange for a more accessible benefit of furloughs. When prison virtually reconstitutes society on the outside down to the smallest detail, the fear of being forever excluded from the free world emerges.

Marriage encounters as seen by legislators

Little by little, the idea of softening the rupture caused by confinement is gaining ground in democracies[274]. Several solutions are envisaged, according to a more or less ambitious desire, ranging from the satisfaction of sexual needs, to the meeting envisaged from a family and emotional point of view. The objective of conjugal encounters alternates between a desire to "serenize" the time spent in detention, so as to facilitate the day-to-day management of confinement, and the ambition to pave the way for a reintegration process, by limiting the

---

273. FOUCAULT (Michel), *op. cit.* p. 133.
274. Back in the 1980s, the French Minister of Justice, Robert Badinter, had already initiated the project for a conjugal dating service.

effects of de-socialization, through the implementation of a policy of maintaining family ties.

The existence of European texts is no stranger to the awareness of the need for change in the area of conjugal encounters. In 1988, the European Commission of Human Rights informed the French government that "it is essential to respect for family life that the prison administration should help prisoners to maintain contact with their immediate family"[275]. In the wake of numerous reports on the particularly critical state of prisons in France, and in view of the trend towards longer sentences, the need for reform has become unavoidable.

Project genesis and borrowings from foreign systems

The prison administration has an obligation to enforce the prerogatives defined and voted by the legislator. Any new right is an additional commitment, with a heavy financial, human and organizational cost, not to mention the responsibilities incumbent on supervisory staff. Authorized and organized sexual relations must be conducted with respect for the human person, at the risk of making the prison administration legally and financially liable for any excesses that result in damage. This is one of the arguments put forward to explain the timidity and inertia of change.

Hispanic countries were undoubtedly the first to recognize the need not to deprive prisoners of sexual relations. Spain and many other Latin American countries, for example, have a long tradition of creating intimate, unsupervised areas where prisoners can have carnal encounters with their partners. These visiting rooms are known as *"sex rooms"*. They usually consist of a room with a bed, a table, two chairs and sanitary

---

275. European Commission of Human Rights, March 12 1990, *Ali Raymond OUINAS v. France*, decision no. 13756/88.

facilities. Both the location and the duration of the visit are unabashedly sexual. Given the fears of the French field, the major drawback lies in the questions of dignity associated with explicitly organizing the sexuality of individuals. The director of the La Plata prison in Argentina explains that this device quickly became commonplace, with no prejudice expressed either on the part of the prison administration, or on the part of the inmates or their spouses.

The Canadian system, on which France based its UVF program, is more elaborate. It involves family gatherings in pavilions called *roulottes*[276], sometimes lasting several days. The aim is to recreate a family life close to that of the outside world, combining emotions and sensuality, and possibly including the presence of children. An evaluation of the program highlighted the shared satisfaction of prison staff and inmates alike, with the demonstration that maintaining family ties is particularly beneficial in terms of rehabilitation objectives. The right to sexuality is not the official foundation of this evolution, even if it is an implicit cornerstone. Although situations of conjugal violence have been noted, it seems that, naturally, the conditions outside the prison are sufficiently reconstituted for prisoners and their spouses alike to experience this *oasis of reunion*, sheltered from the gaze of prison guards, as an opportune moment, an irreplaceable episode, with no equivalent during detention.

Sexual visiting rooms, or other UVFs, attest to the recognition of scxual needs in the lives of inmates. They also recognize the iniquity of incarceration for prisoners' spouses. This development is in line

---

276. Inmates serving sentences of more than two years are required to use the trailers every two months. The duration can vary between two and seventy-two hours. This system was developed from an experiment carried out between 1980 and 1983. Given the satisfactory results shared by all those involved in prison life, the system was extended.

with what the European Committee against Torture and Inhuman and Degrading Treatment (CPT) has been advocating for several years[277]. In the same vein, the Council of Europe adopted a recommendation in 1998, stating that "consideration should be given to giving prisoners the opportunity to meet their sexual partners without visual surveillance during the visit"[278].

In the end, all the misgivings expressed during the interviews appeared to be *a priori* fears, which the comparison with Argentinean prisons helped to allay. The sex rooms there were installed in record time, with limited resources, limiting the space to a converted cell. The Argentinian government was unmoved by the experimental phases that weighed down the decision-making process with incessant *weighing up of* pros and cons, and yet the conclusion was clear: "It would be impossible today to turn back the clock. We even wonder how prisons functioned before *encuentros intimos*[279] existed."[280]

The French system: the choice of family visiting units

Frequently translated as "Family Life Units", given the relational dimension and the fact that the place has no official purpose, UVFs are more ambitious than sex rooms, which are conceived purely as *places for sex*. However, as the saying goes: "if it's *too much, it's too little*", the ambition to *do the best possible* has the disadvantage of delaying the implementation of a process that some people would have liked to see

---

277. Report of the CPT to the Government of the French Republic on the visit to France from October 27 to November 8, 1991.
278. Recommendation No. R(98) of the Committee of Ministers to Member States on the ethical and organizational aspects of health care in prison, adopted on April 8, 1998.
279. Intimate talks in Argentina are invariably referred to as *encuentros íntimos* or *visitas higiénicas*.
280. These are the findings of the director of the La Plata prison in the province of Buenos-Aires.

confirmed years ago. As if it were a question of not contradicting what the prison administration has never wanted to recognize as a prerogative, out of modesty and diplomacy towards prison staff, inmates and a public irritated by the idea of *four-star prisons*, the official language goes out of its way to officially present the UVF as a *family facility*. The Ministry rejects the term *"sex parlor"* and stresses that the stated aim is not to solve the problem of sexuality in prison. Moreover, the name chosen reflects a particular modesty in designating a space whose most innovative features lie in the possibility offered to prisoners to have sexual relations with their partner, on the one hand, and to abstain from the principle of surveillance for a given period of time, on the other.

UVF units are designed as small furnished apartments, comprising a living room and two bedrooms. The space is intended to be a recreation of a *family interior*, understood as a place that favors both the conviviality of the inhabitants, and the intimacy of a couple in a furnished bedroom. Television, sofa, toy and DVD box, in a sober and warm decoration, such are the ingredients of this experience whose vocation consists in positioning the prisoners in conditions similar to the society outside. UVF remains a process of confinement, in which the principle of surveillance is replaced by a temporary reconstitution of intimacy. Imagined many years ago[281], the initial UVF project was announced in the press on December 1st, 1998. It took a long phase of experimentation and conclusions kept secret for a long time before France decided to extend the principle of conjugal encounters, euphemistically referred to as family encounters. The feelings of the inmates benefiting from this new prerogative contradict their own apprehensions as much as the reticence of the prison administration, as this prisoner testifies: "I have

---

281. Under the impetus of the French Minister of Justice, Robert Badinter, in 1984. FAURE (Michaël), "Humaniser pour réinsérer. Le droit à l'intimité en détention", *Le Monde diplomatique*, February 1999.

The love life in detention - controlled otherness -

to admit that this interlude of peace in the brutal universe of the prison world does my head a world of good, and for those who come to visit us it's even better. No more crowded visiting rooms, no more noise, no more waiting, no more stress, no more tension - in short, it's a break where you can rediscover yourself intimately, where you have a little more time to feel, talk and even listen to the silence together."[282]

At the very heart of detention, the UVF system highlights all the issues involved in resocialization in the free world after release. It acts as a process of gradual "re-familiarization" with unsupervised existence, confrontation with chosen otherness, free sharing and tenderness.

Access conditions

Access to the UVF is reserved for permanently sentenced prisoners[283] who cannot benefit from a sentence modification guaranteeing the maintenance of family ties. In other words, only "non-permissible" prisoners, and this is the first criticism of the system. While this limitation may seem sensible from a theoretical point of view, the reality contradicts the rationale behind this precision, insofar as only a small proportion of "permissible" prisoners actually benefit from permission[284]. As a result, the conditions of access to the UVF may be unfair and inappropriate.

The concept of visitors having access to the UVF is a broad one. They may be family members who can prove their family ties, or persons with whom the inmate has a *lasting affective bond*. The reality of this qualification is investigated by the commission in charge of granting visitation permits. In keeping with the principle of non-discrimination

---

282. MANAUD-BENAZERAF (Sylvie), *Les Unités de visites familiales. Nouvelles pratiques, nouveaux liens*, Agen, Cirap, 2006, p. 69.
283. This excludes the prison population.
284. At Val-de-Reuil, for example, in 2007, only 71 out of 430 inmates were granted leave. The prison administration was unable to provide national figures.

on the basis of sexual orientation, the UVF is also open to homosexual couples. Visits are authorized by the prison governor, after consultation with staff, and following interviews with visitors and inmates. The only grounds for refusal are security[285]. The notion of security is also understood in a broad sense. The aim is, of course, to guarantee safety in detention, but also the mental and physical safety of UVF users, who are under the responsibility of the prison administration.

The duration of visits alternates gradually between six and forty-eight hours, depending on the decision of the head of the establishment, and on the request of the persons concerned. Exceptionally, once a year, the UVF may be granted for a period of seventy-two hours. The frequency used in France is quarterly. On the whole, the system chosen by the French legislature is very much inspired by the ambitions of the Canadian system, in terms of space design, frequency and duration, albeit with a thirty-year time lag, which, in view of the pace of future planned installations, attests to persistent policy inertia: of the one hundred and ninety prisons, as of July 1st, 2007, seven were equipped with UVF. And of the nineteen new prisons scheduled for 2012, only seventeen will be equipped[286].

In the UVF, privacy and security are combined while respecting each other. Unlike visiting rooms, there is no direct surveillance. Only outside rounds and external surveillance of the building are carried out by video surveillance. During visits, surveillance staff may enter the UVF, provided they announce themselves beforehand via an internal intercom. Also, at set times and in accordance with internal regulations,

---

285. For information, in 2006, 92% of requests were approved, 5% were postponed and 3% rejected. See BOUGEARD (Nathalie), *Lien social*, no 826, February 1st, 2007.
286. Statement by the Minister of Justice, published in *Libération*, Thursday June 19, 2008.

supervisors enter the studio to check that everything is running smoothly. They often take the pretext of bringing something with them to lessen the effect of *surveillance*.

The official UVF balance sheet

As in all the countries where the experiment has been tried, and against the respective apprehensions of supervisory staff and inmates, the results of the UVF seem to be particularly positive[287]. The director of the Poissy facility concludes: "It's extremely positive for maintaining ties.[288] She also refers to the need to "manage very intense emotions, for both inmates and their families, who for years have often shared only a few hours of visiting time". Individuals relearn autonomy in the most basic personal behaviors. Family relationships are maintained, and a whole range of existential benefits are derived from reunions, confrontations with otherness, forgetting about incarceration and erasing surveillance. These benefits compensate for the deficiencies imposed by solitary sexuality and the violence of a monosexual world of excitement.

The UVF system represents recognized progress, benefiting prisoners, their families and supervisory staff. The rehabilitation project is encouraged by the reduction in desocialization. However, whatever the material conditions, the UVF remains intrinsically linked to the punitive system, instrumentalized to satisfy the respective interests of the two social groups that make up prison society. The first novelty of UVF is the implicit yet official recognition of the pathogenic effects of confinement. The second novelty is the emphasis placed on a common interest between the prison administration and the inmate population,

---

287. The first report on the UVF experiment is classified as a *non-disclosable document*. See RAMBOURG (Cécile), *L'Expérimentation des UEVF au CP de Rennes*, Agen, École nationale d'administration pénitentiaire, 2005-2006. A second assessment was published: MANAUD-BENAZERAF (Sylvie), *op. cit.*
288. *Le Figaro*, June 30, 2006.

with a view to the future. The effects of this revolution in the way we redefine the power to punish are numerous. It's a temporary and temporary abandonment of the panoptic principle that had previously governed the institution. The UVF transforms the role of warders, and consequently the way in which inmates view these individuals, whose function is no longer limited to guarding. In this respect, Sylvie Manaud-Benazeraf notes[289] that the recognition of the need for reunions, and the staging of these encounters, have a notoriously pacifying effect within the prison. It is also a remedy for the daily violence exacerbated by monosexual confinement and the deprivation of otherness.

The UVF overturns the roles assigned to prison staff. Prison wardens are no longer simply guards, but are valued in a role akin to that of a social worker. Prisoners are no longer reduced to their offenses, and regain a form of autonomy that they govern momentarily sheltered from the surveillance mechanism[290]. By bringing the outside in, UVFs breathe life into a population maintained in existential lethargy. Prison thus loses some of its status as a social coffin[291] in the words of Michel Onfray. All the conclusions drawn from UVF experiments point to benefits that are a response to the consequences of sexual deprivation. The new-found otherness enables prisoners to reposition themselves as sexual actors in their own existence, interceding in the existence of others. As opposed to any virtuality, the encounter with the other in the conditions offered by reunion favours the temporary suspension of the feeling of the sentence experienced as a "period of total exile from life"[292]. The intermittent nature of UVFs thus alleviates the

---

289. MANAUD-BENAZERAF (Sylvie), *op. cit.* p. 70.
290. See ALVAREZ (Josefina), "Chronique de l'exécution des peines", *Revue de sciences criminelles et de droit pénal comparé*, Paris, July-September 2006, p. 658.
291. ONFRAY (Michel), *9 m²*, Paris, Le Cadratin/Acte Sud, 2006, p. 87.
292. GOFFMAN (Erving), *op. cit.* p. 113.

The love life in detention - controlled otherness -

duration of long sentences, providing an antidote to the feeling of infinite confinement.

Of course, there is room for criticism. In the interests of empowerment, it has been decided to make inmates financially responsible for hosting their relatives. This educational measure is not without its problems for indigent inmates, for whom the prison administration is unable to provide work. Under certain conditions, the UVF can appear unfair when the meeting of relatives is conditional on purchasing power, which is particularly problematic within the prison walls. On the other hand, among all the apprehensions that inmates may have beforehand, there is one that has not been dispelled by the UVF experiment. This is the fear that this system will tend to make people forget that confinement is theoretically recommended as an exceptional measure. While the theoretical will to do so is likely to appease international criticism of France's lag in respecting the dignity of detainees, these intentions lose some of their credibility when we observe the timidity of the system in relation to actual needs.

THE THWARTED AMBITIONS OF REINTEGRATION

Imprisonment, constant humiliation and the recognition that imprisoned individuals are often victims of a society reluctant to tolerate differences or destructive experiences, make prison an instrument of justice often perceived as unfair and inappropriate. It has to be said that the challenges facing the prison administration are particularly complex. Caught in the vice of European regulations, the Code of Criminal Procedure, technical and ideological developments in society, and public policies on justice and repression, prison officials are regularly forced to give pragmatic priority to ideology or the *strict* application of the law. The constraint of confinement generates forms of resistance commensurate with the authoritarian power it represents. Prison is a reminder that illegality and disobedience have no other scale of reference and motivation than the number of prohibitions formulated. This repressive institution bears witness to the limits of the very principle of repression, which induces resistance to order, and feeds the organization of disorder and disobedience, conceived as so many illegalisms enabling one to survive domination. Prison raises the question of the human species' capacity to be tamed, and the survival issues that arise in maintaining physical and mental integrity. In this case, sexuality and the desire for privacy are mechanisms for safeguarding this integrity.

The thwarted ambitions of reintegration

This study began with the question raised by the paradox between the undisputed certainty of the importance of sexuality to the wholeness of beings, on the one hand, and the manifest inertia regarding the effective recognition of a right to intimacy in detention, on the other. In the words of Maurice Godelier[293], sexuality is "always something other than itself", and in the context of *long-sentence* incarceration, it enables us to describe social realities on the borders of affective and sensual dimensions.

In the face of this lack of legislation on sexual matters, there is a notorious lack of interest in prison policies. By action and omission, the management of sexual issues in prisons clearly prioritizes the desire to punish over the desire to rehabilitate. Can the prison administration's stated ambition of resocialization be reconciled with the punitive objective that prevailed in the original concept of confinement? What is the face of an institution whose remit seems so contradictory? It's clear that prison is defined more by its paradoxes than by its successes. If it has always lacked credibility, it's probably because it has never considered respectability a priority, except perhaps today with the advent of UVF. The emergence of an interest in the right to privacy is one of the main reasons why democracies have made a major shift in their conception of punishment. The choice of the UVF in France, as much as the other systems put in place in other countries, is the expression of an observation highlighting the dangers and inefficiency of global coercion as envisaged in prison confinement. It's not so much a questioning of the legitimacy of the power to punish as a criticism of the counter-productive side-effects of the disruptive effect of relegation and isolation. By trying too hard to contrast inside and outside, landmarks are lost, vengeance feeds, and violence compensates for yawning

---

293. GODELIER (Maurice), "La sexualité est autre chose qu'elle-même", *Esprit*, March-April 2001, p. 96.

lacks of otherness and self-esteem. Prison's excessive desire to deprive individuals of such essential existential dimensions as the freedom of sensual and emotional encounters with otherness means that, through a global asceticism, the experience of imprisonment is reduced to a form diametrically opposed to that of the outside world. Individual survival mechanisms are organized around a visceral need to be, to exist, to be recognized as a singular entity with an identity space in society.

The consequences of imprisonment are not neutral for society on the outside. Following feelings of injustice in the face of suffering that degrades more than it repairs, prison arouses hatred, anger and vengeance towards society, in the very place where it should be *calming* a social climate based on respect for people, property and the law. This regime seems to forget that one day, perhaps, one day without doubt, prisoners will have to leave the institution, to reintegrate a society in which the issue of their *place* remains fundamental. Prisoners survive with a hatred that is matched only by the deconstruction of their personalities over the years. Because it is perceived as unjust and ill-adapted to the variety of delinquency profiles, because it gives precedence to ostracism and punishment over any ambition for rehabilitation, because it underlines social and cultural inequalities, the institution operates a transfer of vengeance between the society on the outside, which demands order and the atonement of faults, and the society on the inside, which leaves this *school of delinquency* with a hatred equalled only by the degradation suffered. This observation is reminiscent of Gresham Sykes' conclusions[294] about American high-security prisons, as well as those of Édouard Desprez[295] in 1868.

---

294. SYKES (Gresham), *The Society of Captives. A Study of a Maximum Security Prison*, translated from the English by Arnaud Gaillard, Princeton (N.J.), Princeton University Press, 1958, p. 22.
295. DESPREZ (Édouard), *De l'abolition de l'emprisonnement*, Paris, Dentu, 1868, p. 40.

The thwarted ambitions of reintegration

The experience of sexuality in the prison environment also reminds us that the mechanisms of constraint and contradiction of satisfactions generate resistance. Even if the majority of inmates recognize prison as an inescapable institution, it is often accepted more as a punishment for other people's delinquency than for their own. Finally, on various scales, the illegal acts and disobedience that take place in prison are not far removed from behavior outside. On the contrary, they reflect an exact echo of it, demonstrating a common humanity that it would be pointless to divide along Manichean lines.

Chapter 1
The paradox of body discipline

"As Foucault writes, sexuality is not what power is afraid of, but what power is exercised through: sexual liberation, inscribed in relations of power, would not so much be 'the uncovering of secret truths about oneself or one's desire, as an element in the process of defining and constructing desire'."[296]

Whether in terms of prohibition or authorization, sexuality or the right to sexuality is *conspicuous by its absence* in all the legislative and regulatory documents governing prisons. Prohibition is metaphorized behind evocations of *modesty* and *obscenity*, while the organization of couple relationships, within the UVF, is evoked behind objectives of maintaining family ties. Unquestionably, sexuality belongs to the intimate sphere of the individual. Perhaps this is another reason why the legislator does not claim the legitimacy of officially and expressly organizing the conditions of practice. And yet, under the surface, the prison system, in its essence and in the exceptions it allows itself, organizes a veritable discipline of bodies and pleasures. There is a clear contrast between what cannot be mentioned, and the power actually exercised.

---

296. Daoust (Valérie), *op. cit.* p. 181.

Whatever the historical, legal or sociological justifications for this state of affairs, this contradiction is the first in a series of paradoxes governing the prison condition. It's as if the very principle of confinement could not rigorously obey a rational project, so much does it upset the condition of the human species, and so much does it strive to reconcile the irreconcilable.

Prison authority is gradually moving from an imperative regime to a fluctuating one, which loses and lulls claims into a set of constructed paradoxes, in which new prerogatives, offered to some, are a disguised way of establishing, for others, a form of unilateral power of domination. The gradual penetration of humanist virtues within the prison is not to the detriment of the institution's authority, which remains unchallenged because it is indisputable. Questions of sexuality are at the heart of this evolution in the power of the prison administration. Because the effectiveness of the ban on sexual relations is an illusion, the management of imprisonment, in terms of sexuality, obeys a series of conjunctural paradoxes that navigate between a disciplinary will and the impossibility of controlling the unmanageable. Since authority to prohibit sexual relations cannot be conceived as radically effective, power is discretionary and is exercised under the uncertainty of disciplinary sanctions. Philippe Combessie has shown that the control of pleasures is not so much a matter for *general*, security-oriented *power*, as for the mechanisms of "interstitial powers"[297], which are lodged in the specific features of prison organization, or are deduced from the contingencies of confinement.

Beyond the embodiment of power, the elaboration of paradoxical situations, between radicality and the fluctuation of prohibitions,

---

297. COMBESSIE (Philippe), *op. cit.* p. 140.

constitutes a measure of domination, signifying to individuals that they cannot have recourse to a rational process to argue, defend themselves or contest their submission. Beyond the disciplinary system based on the organization of "ordered multiplicities" referred to by Foucault[298], the prison articulates its authority around paradoxes, unquestionable because they are unpredictable, irrational and random. Particularly in sexual matters, the coherence of the expected order is obtained from the incoherence of an instrumentalized and maintained disorder. This conclusion echoes those of Michel Foucault when he describes the mechanisms of discipline behind the analysis of a "microphysics of power". It's a combination of circumstances and processes that enable some to dominate others, in the service of personal, institutional or state power. In all cases, the pretext of standardizing behavior allows the staging of hierarchical and disciplinary relationships that establish coercion legitimized by disobedience. Under prison conditions, sexuality is sociologically objectified and politically rationalized, in a measured process of repression and domination.

---

298. Foucault (Michel), *op. cit.* p. 149.

Chapter 2
From restraining bodies to controlling the senses and pleasures

Always contested, decried and criticized for its inadequacies, injustice and counter-productivity, prison remains, in our democratic societies, the priority instrument of the penal system, in defiance of European penitentiary rules, which reiterate that "no one may be deprived of his or her liberty, unless such deprivation of liberty constitutes a measure of last resort and is in accordance with procedures defined by law"[299]. The institution is intended to be coercive as a deterrent, to be redemptive, to satisfy society's *a priori desire for* defensive vengeance. Far from the initial definition of a prison as a place where the freedom to come and go is denied, the prison regime is nurtured by a punitive austerity that is combined with a wide range of deprivations. Sexuality, whether restricted or organized, is a reminder that the coercive mechanism of prison is first and foremost founded on a principle of restriction. Whether it's the restriction of space, encounters, opportunities, actions or pleasures, prison systematizes the organization of a *life of too little* and an *existence of lack*.

---

299. Council of Europe Recommendation no. 2006-2, January 11, 2006. Although recommendations are not legally binding, the European Court of Human Rights is increasingly using them as a basis for binding judgments.

Every attempt to humanize the prison institution comes up against the desires of a society that expects the principle of obedience to the law to derive from the principle of confinement. Prison is not just a punishment for an offence, it must also be a threat in everyone's mind. For this reason, any new provision in favor of the rights of detainees must be accompanied by a mechanism that enables the prison authorities to *maintain control* while remaining a deterrent.

In its current form, control of sexuality is based on a combination of prohibition and compensation. In its future form, with the development of the UVF, control of sexuality is organized around a set of relative authorizations, whose final authority and the circumstances that inspire it remain at the discretion of the prison administration. The coercion of sexual practices, disregarding the reality of needs, attests to a desire to maintain dissatisfaction during detention. The prison administration administers desire just as the law requires it to administer freedom. Controlling the sexuality of detainees is part and parcel of the totalizing aspects of the penitentiary institution, when it reduces offenders to *puppets* whose existence is appropriated in its most intimate aspects. This is the meaning of corporal punishment, described by Michel Foucault as inescapable "to a certain extent", as opposed to the uselessness of punishment that is merely incorporeal[300]. And yet, the punishment thus envisaged goes beyond the body itself, to reach individuals at the very heart of their humanity, around questions of intimacy, self-esteem, autonomy and freedom.

At a time when physical integrity is protected by humanist concepts and legal provisions, the body can no longer be objectified or punished as it once was. The constraint exerted by the authority of the prison admi-

---

300. Foucault (Michel), *op. cit.* pp. 21-22 and 124.

nistration must progressively be applied to a less controllable domain, with at least equivalent coercive effectiveness. From a constraint of the mind deduced from the constraint of bodies, we have now moved on to a more abstract constraint deduced from the control of the senses and pleasures. In the economy of a punishment based on the sole principle of deprivation of liberty, the physical body, which can no longer be reached by means of torments now prohibited, is subjected to deprivations intimately combined with psychic constraints. Control of the body has gradually been replaced by control of the senses. The authority of the prison administration manifests itself and is maintained through castration mechanisms that fragment the individuals locked up, through marked or symbolic control of what belongs to the intimate. These processes entrench a culture of fear, sometimes embodied in paranoid behavior defining all otherness as a potential enemy, sometimes in submission to authoritarian, omnipresent discipline.

Isolation, as understood in the context of relegation, is the paradigm of an institution whose ambition is to restore the notion of respect for others, while at the same time organizing an amputation of the other. Initially private, otherness is sporadically restored, under controlled conditions, in the visiting rooms and, more generously, in the still embryonic UVF system. This situation is a reminder that too much constraint can lead to destruction. The management of sexual issues is part of a more general process of constraint, which does not allow for serenity or peace of mind, and affects both physical and psychological integrity.

The control of pleasures and the acceptance of violence, analyzed in detention as the defense of the identity of fragmented individualities, represent two artifacts of power. The punitive system of the prison comes close to the disciplinary conception of religions when they organize mechanisms of submission and obedience based on the control of pleasures. In the same way, it is by means of an external entity to which individual autonomies are devolved, voluntarily or involuntarily, that privative authority is underpinned by notions of punishment, fault and guilt, undoubtedly arousing more incomprehension and hatred than redemptive efficacy.

The control of pleasures through control, denunciation, surveillance and confession, are all manifestations of a power that exults in prison. Whether ideological, scientific, political or religious, the control of pleasure is an expression of power that serves the control of the masses. It's not so much the origin of the ban that's important. Above all, it's the fear of what the human mass would become without prohibitions that motivates the organization of an order, as opposed to a presumed chaos. Whether we're talking about behavior, practice, orientation or desire, sexuality is widely regarded in society as a potentially destabilizing factor, likely to downgrade the *fundamentals* embodied in order, obedience, possession and a whole cohort of earthly rationalities that posit the present day as a prelude to the interests of tomorrow. This fear of chaos is instrumentalized in the elaboration of an economy of powers that legitimizes authority, both in essence and in practice, in order to satisfy the objectives of prosperity.

The confinement of *long sentences subjects people*'s lives to a form of lethargy of the body, mind and social position of the individual. When it doesn't limit itself to deprivation of liberty, when it doesn't do everything possible to erase as far as possible this rupture between the outside and the inside, prison simulates, over the years, a symbolic, watered-down capital punishment, of which it represents a *politically correct* version in terms of contemporary standards of fundamental rights. Sexuality in prison reveals the slow degradation of individuals until their psychological and social death. Bodies wither away, and the relationship with otherness makes the outside world seem like unfamiliar territory. The hatred of an oppressive, totalizing system, which leads to a loss of self-esteem, can only lead to chain reactions that dangerously compromise the prospects of reintegration. This conclusion on the flawed relationship with otherness corroborates the work of Robert M. Lindner[301]; the other is the mirror of "who we are" and "how we love ourselves". However, as release approaches, the question of reintegration becomes a major issue, from an individual point of view for the inmates in terms of managing their respective lives, and from a collective point of view for the society outside that will welcome them, or not, upon release. Paul Schilder states that "the death instinct becomes effectively destructive when it is not neutralized by a sufficient supply of libido"[302]. Other authors[303] speak of a progressive castration, synonymous with a life that slowly but surely slips away, in the manner of a psychic and social lobotomy. Confinement thus considered reminds us that the punitive principle cannot be understood without an aggregation of sufferings, designed to establish a mechanism of domination whose intensity is proportional to the desire to disobey. These often respond to the echo of a political desire to normalize behavior.

---

301. LINDNER (Robert M.), *Sex in Prison*, translated by Arnaud Gaillard, Fall, Complex, 1951, p. 72.
302. SCHILDER (Paul), *op. cit.* p. 141.
303. Including Antoinette Chauvenet, Françoise Orlic, Georges Benguigui, Jacques Lesage de La Haye, François Danet, Sophie Ferrucci, Alain Monnereau, Paul Schilder, Simone Buffard, Bruno Bettelheim, Daniel Welzer-Lang, Michaël Faure, Lilian Mathieu, Dominique Lhuilier, Luc Ridel, Aldona Simonpietri, Claude Veil.

Chapter 3
Guilt and the mechanisms
of regression-degradation-humiliation

The experience of sexuality in the prison environment highlights the processes of humiliation resulting from the many forms of violence generated by imprisonment. Imprisonment is based on these mechanisms of degradation, in which the punishment incurred is a daily reminder of the guilt of the offence committed. It is in this sense that the deprivations organized by the prison come into play. Punishment for illegality stigmatizes offenders in their failure to respect irreproachable behavior. The loss of dignity begins with the commission of offences and, when the institution doesn't take it upon itself to point this out, inmates organize themselves among themselves, to "inter-degrade" based on acts that most often have sexual connotations.

The meticulousness of psychic torments in the alcove of the conscious and unconscious is a discreet but nonetheless manifest destructuring of these offending individuals. With its vocation to punish evil, and based on a sexuality that is sometimes prohibited or repressed, sometimes restrictively organized, prison organizes a regression of individuals by depriving them of the attributes of autonomy that characterize adult life. Offenses represent a misuse of freedom and autonomy. Punishment then strives to organize the regression of a detained population that has confessed, on the outside, its inability to use freedom in compliance with standards.

The exacerbation of violence in detention is both the cause and consequence of feelings of humiliation. More than anywhere else, the collective otherness experienced here predates individual identities. Sometimes stripped of their adult status, sometimes reduced to prison numbers or offenses, inmates develop survival behaviors, in a process that is both defensive against the hostility of a reconstituted micro-society, and existential against the social death provoked by the totalizing stakes of a leveling institution.

The experience of sexuality in detention raises questions about the humanity of individuals deprived of freedom and autonomy, whose existence is reduced to a narcissistic relationship in masturbations weaned from a chosen otherness. Through these daily deprivations that touch on intimacy, society signifies to individuals the illegitimacy of their freedom outside. Regressive mechanisms are then born of the many degrading behaviors that are expressed as coping and compensatory mechanisms. Simone Buffard describes these numerous psychic and social destructurations in this way, pointing out that the worst is not yet over until the regressions are definitive[304]. The Manichean viewpoint of prison staff as the wilful perpetrators of these daily humiliations is erroneous. Prison administration staff are entrusted with a custodial mission, subject to potential hierarchical control, in the exercise of a profession with sometimes summary but always real responsibilities. This analysis does not rule out the existence of excesses, which are certainly all too frequent, but the exception does

---

304. BUFFARD (Simone), *op. cit.* p. 44.

not make the rule. As a result, the institution's dangerousness is not so much attributable to its players as to the very principle of authoritarian confinement that governs it.

Humiliation is organized around intermittent recognition of sexual needs. On the one hand, unsatisfied libido is uniformly described as a source of violence. On the other, pornography is disseminated, homosexuality is de facto encouraged, then repressed, and carnal exchanges in visiting rooms are randomly made possible[305]. In this situation of uncertainty, sexual practices are carried out in degrading circumstances, with the fear of being caught, the threat of disciplinary action, and intimacy subverted by the collective. The humiliations thus experienced are closely linked to the certainty that inmates can have, of being globally subject to the prison administration, which alone is free to grant clemency, indulgence, organize the circumstances of the practices, and tomorrow, to formulate its authorization. In all cases, the prison emphasizes to *inmates* that it remains sovereign. Therein lies the credibility of its supreme authority in the process of legal punishment, and it is through the gratifying concept of Justice that it legitimizes its existence and its structural imperfections.

---

305. See also MONTANDON (Cléopâtre) and CUETTAZ (Bernard), *op. cit.*, p. 141.

Chapter 4
Sexual deprivation, otherness deprivation and desocialization

Undoubtedly, imprisonment provokes a rupture from which existences will organize themselves into economies of survival, which are nothing other than forms of adaptation, whose objective is to maintain the integrity of the self. Over the course of long sentences, the deprivation of sexual relations is tantamount to the compression of desires which, because they can no longer be expressed, gradually lead to the disappearance of the feeling of existence. Prison society, made up of the forced amalgamation of these individualities in need, feeds on compensatory processes that find their incarnation in mechanisms of violence for some and perversion for others. Whether it's a question of violence turned against oneself, violence against others, or the development of a culture of hatred cleverly nurtured over the years against the institution and society that mandates it, prison very often locks up delinquents and sets free *desocialized wild beasts*.

The desire to restrict sexual relations too much means that it is not so much the notion of orgasmic pleasure that is lacking, but rather the otherness that is indispensable to the construction of social being. For not content with organizing a geographical ostracism by relegating individuals to the confines of its walls, the contemporary prison deprives individuals of the attributes that enable them to recognize themselves through otherness. The lack of sexuality is not so much the lack of sexual pleasure or the consumption of what hormones encourage, but rather the feeling of no longer existing without a relationship of desire, seduction, sex and shared pleasure.

In detention, this other that is so lacking represents the lack of an indispensable ingredient for the completeness of beings. The detainee population is confronted with the constraint of a solitude that replaces the lost existence of otherness on the outside. The encounter with the desire and body of this other, who cannot be chosen, gives way to an inert solitude, deceived by the virtuality of fantasized excitements. Coping mechanisms develop in an attempt to respond to the lack of the other, to the "recovery" of the self, to the satisfaction of pleasure and the feeling of completeness. The monosexual specificity of confinement inevitably leads prisoners to develop homosexual practices, consented to or undergone as the case may be, in an attempt to compensate for the missing otherness of another gender. These sexual practices give rise to relationships of interest and domination, violence and possession, underlining the close and inescapable link between sexuality and power. Beyond the satisfaction of libidinal impulses, prison homosexuality authorizes a sexuality in which otherness reclaims its rights. And yet, in many situations, these sexual practices are consented to only on the assumption of the fantasized substitution of a body, whose gender is made to disappear, the better to inhabit it with a materialized virtuality. In all cases, regardless of consent, male homosexuality raises issues of identity that have a direct impact on self-esteem. *Egos* are sometimes damaged, leading to narcissistic wounds that can only find an outlet in constant homophobia, and violence that underlines the survival of masculinity in the men's prison. Prisoners play a daily game of evaluation and *perpetual challenge*, ensuring in the eyes of others, and in their own eyes, the survival of a *dominant phallus.* The *masculine aura* depends on this feeling of power, which is never so acquired as in the exercise of a sexuality in which the phallus exults, through its rectitude and capacity to penetrate, in the power of its holder's identity.

In stark contrast, the women inmates do not suffer any identity disturbances as a result of their homosexual practices. In response to a mortifying solitude, and out of a concern for tenderness, attentiveness and closeness, both sentimental and carnal, relationships are formed between women, with a lightness matched only by the vehemence of male behavior in such situations. As the years go by, however, mono-sexual confinement blurs the significance of autonomous encounters with the other gender. In this sense, confinement and the distortion of the relationship to otherness, combined with mechanisms of continual frustration, constitute a particularly de-socializing environment. Prison unlearns the ability to live together by exacerbating defense mechanisms and violence. The solitude of sexual practices and the virtuality of arousal objects gradually distort our appreciation of this *similar other* who is not ourselves.

The lack of otherness must be compensated for in detention, not only by solitary sexual activity, supported by widespread pornography, but also and above all by techniques for re-appropriating the self. Sport, body maintenance understood as both an ornamental and a protective envelope, and discourses that bring into virtual existence what no longer exists factually, are all ways of reconstituting the missing gaze of a *desired* and *desired otherness.* But these substitutes have their limits. While *talking about sex* stamps individuals as sexed and therefore existing beings, in all cases, talking is not acting. What we see in men is an identity wound that can only be soothed by expressions of virilizing violence, like a catharsis that needs to be repeated because it proves so ineffective. Women experience this absence of shared desire as an abandonment that reduces their lives to a form of dehumanized wandering, coloring the years of imprisonment with an emptiness that leaves a lasting impression of being nothing. The extension of the use of the UVF will undoubtedly gradually correct this discrepancy caused by confinement. By authorizing affective encounters and the sexual dimension, virtualized compensations will be attenuated in favor of the *possibilities* that justice now intends to authorize, propose and control. For human beings, it's a question of recovering the capacity to give and receive, which attests to the personal sensation of existing and the recognition by otherness of one's own *quality of existing*.

However, this new liberality is intended to respond more to a sexual need viewed from the physiological angle, than to the restoration of social ties, raising the question of *one's place* in the group, based on chosen and controlled occurrences[306]. UVF represents a response to sexuality understood in a rational way, and neglects irrational dimensions such as free access to the occurrence of practices, in spatio-temporal conditions that make affective and sexual encounters privileged rendezvous, between two free and consenting actors, fully masters of the destiny of their intimacy. Because in prison, it's the *autonomous being* that is stifled by detention, and while UVFs tend to reconstitute the circumstances that enable detainees to rediscover their singularity when encountering a partner, this autonomy is suspended from conditions that only the prison administration masters. The autonomy that is sporadically granted is therefore never acquired.

---

306. See also Welzer-Lang (Daniel) and Mathieu (Lilian), "Des significations de la sexualité en milieu carcéral", *Les Cahiers de la sécurité intérieure*, "Prisons en société", no. 31, Paris, 1998, p. 228.

The thwarted ambitions of reintegration

Chapter 5
Minimal characterization of living organisms

Like many situations of deprivation, the institution implicitly defines the parameters that characterize life. Prison is experienced as an institution that steals life, leaving only the satisfaction of essential physiological survival, with no specifically human dimension and no social reference point. The constitutive elements of survival, and therefore of legally defined life, are organized around the physical body, understood as the primordial entity for identifying individuals and recognizing the *fact of existing*. In prison, the existence of individuals is suspended by a definition of the living that reduces the human species to the functioning of organs according to medically recognized criteria. The prison administration is responsible for guarding individuals within a fortress whose walls represent the concrete dimension, and in which discipline and deprivation represent the abstract dimension. The *penitentiary's* role in the execution of criminal justice is based on its obligation to ensure that detainees survive the temporary sentence of imprisonment. This survival is essentially and primarily envisaged in terms of the survival of the bodily envelope, conceived as a coordinated association of organs.

In prison, the living is characterized above all by the physical mechanics of bodies, according to a hierarchy that places the concrete dimension of the physical far ahead of the abstractions represented by the mind, feelings and social existence. This conception is a denial of the completeness of existence, and of the infinitely complex notions presiding over the more or less rational alchemy that defines man, between the *material* and the *immaterial,* the *concrete* and the *abstract,* the *physical* and the *mental,* the *body* and the *spirit, desires* and *power.* Prison discards the psychoanalytical dimensions that establish an analogy between *libido* and *life drive,* between *desire* and *existing.* The only space of freedom in which resistance can develop lies in the immateriality of thoughts.

An analysis of the experience of sexuality in prison highlights the concept of *social death,* understood as a different kind of finitude, which runs counter to what rehabilitation can represent. If release consists in putting an end to a situation of temporary relegation, what meaning can be given to this perspective when existential reference points have been lost, self-esteem devalued, and when the deprivation and violence accumulated during long sentences have given way to a hatred of the institution and the entire society that mandates it?

However, there have been some positive developments. Significant investment is being made in psychological care. But if despair, prescriptions for psychotropic drugs and inadequate financial and human resources in the face of a particularly destabilized penal population are anything to go by, mental well-being in prison - understood here as an argument for possible reintegration - is definitely not a priority.

If the notion of *manifest torture* has now disappeared, to make way for a prison that is increasingly *humanized*[307], punishment is now conceived at the cost of a coexistence of *good humanist sentiments,*

---

307. See also VEIL (Claude) and LHUILIER (Dominique), (ed.), *op. cit.,* p. 9.

combined with the indispensable power of an institution that believes it disqualifies its existence as soon as it loses in authority what it grants in prerogatives. Yet, under the argument that *civilization is advancing* at the same pace as the legitimization of punishment is receding, it is probably pragmatism that will triumph in the evolution of punitive systems. That's *only* if, one day, society tires of the ineffectiveness of an institution in promoting social peace, or worse still, of the danger posed to a free society by the often irreparable degradation suffered by prisoners during long sentences.

Chapter 6
Incipient recognition of the right to privacy

The organization of conjugal encounters during detention raises the question of the well-being of detainees. This development contrasts with the preoccupations of the 19th century[308]. The emergence of societal concern for the prison population has historically occurred with a significant time lag compared to *society on the* outside. When it comes to penal policy, France is particularly fierce about changing the mechanisms of punishment. The country's penitentiaries are in a state of disrepair, overcrowding is on the increase, and repressive policies are exacerbating the situation, while deprivation of liberty is used almost exclusively as a penal sanction. And yet, "it is in the collective interest that prison should make social reintegration possible. Security is not just about repression, it's also about respect and solidarity"[309].

If civil society is once again particularly mobilized to bring about change in the prison institution, it is likely that the militant energy developed by many organizations is limited to the indispensable

---

308. See Leonard (J.), "Les médecins des prisons", *in* Petit (Jacques-Guy), (ed.), *La Prison, le bagne et l'histoire*, Genève, Librairie des Méridiens, 1984, p. 191.
309. Gil-Robles (Álvaro), European Commissioner for Human Rights, *Libération*, September 22, 2005.

The thwarted ambitions of reintegration

behaviors of resistance, observation and denunciation. The slow pace of change is mainly due to the need for alignment with other European countries, encouraged by provisions that are not binding, but which associations and NGOs can use to put pressure on public authorities.

The constant ambition of reformers of all eras has been to bring *society into the prison*. The choice is between a range of measures to promote reintegration, which would be as many latitudes developed to the detriment of a power to punish hitherto envisaged from the angle of an *aggregate of suffering* to be inflicted. Bringing the outside in is the most frequent recommendation of institutional reformers, as if, from a theoretical point of view, prisons were regularly criticized for what defines them: the thickness and impermeability of their walls. It's also as if this bitter observation is without appeal: *confinement is dangerous for society and harmful for the individuals held there*. This paradox of an institution defined by remoteness and confinement is only the first in a long series of contradictions governing the experience of sexuality in detention. The institution finds itself faced with the impossible task of reconciling a degrading punitive system, which generates social hatred, with a stated ambition for resocialization. As a result, the challenge facing prisons today is to resocialize the very people they de-socialize. This is the contradictory basis of its existence in a democracy. Any change now envisaged can only be an imperfect compromise on the permeability of these walls, which protect in the short term what they destroy in the long term.

By definition, prison is a liberticidal device, but the law fails to define or respect the scope of acceptable legal exceptions. The deprivation of *freedom of movement* is the foundation of incarceration. However, because the process of confinement is not without questioning a certain number of situations, many other exceptions are deduced, imposed and likely to argue an indisputable disciplinary mechanism. Between decades of forbidden conjugal sexuality, and the gradual advent of conjugal encounters, it would be hard not to underline a notable evolution in the coercion of bodies and minds, which confinement is intended to organize. However, whether we're talking about the total deprivation of sexuality, or the dispossession of the occurrence of carnal encounters to the benefit of an organization external to the individuals concerned, such as UVFs and other sexual visiting rooms, the intrusion of the power of the prison administration into the organization of intimacy is not neutral. It is a damaging factor, not only for the psyche of those incarcerated, but also for their ability to be resocialized.

Between a *fundamental need* and an *inalienable right*, sexual practices remain in the realm of the intimate, without being subject to a protective or negotiable legal denomination. The entire legal argument surrounding sexual relations is based on the notion of consent, understood as free and informed. Our societies protect sexuality as a positive, voluntary act. On the other hand, nothing defines the abstraction of need, nor guarantees the autonomy of practices. It's as if the question of consent only governed sexual relations in terms of physical contact, without the law ever enshrining the individual freedom of choice of practices, behind the right to control one's own body.

It is often pragmatic arguments that have made it possible to advance measures previously defended by militancy. When it comes to changing prison conditions, believing in the victory of ideologies is tantamount to confronting a nagging impatience. UVFs are slowly being introduced by a government which knows that this grant of pleasure will become essential to justify the incarceration to which society is increasingly resorting, and to curb potential revolt movements which cannot be silenced indefinitely with psychotropic prescriptions or increasingly severe disci-

303

plinary techniques[310]. *Letting go does* not mean resolving a situation. What's more, the new prerogative offered by UVF is a new instrument of the totalizing power of prisons and the policies that instrumentalize their function. This *authorization of sexuality*, left to the more or less marked discretion of the prison administration, is not seen today as the recognition of a truly inalienable and fundamental right to intimacy. It would have been illusory to hope, under the ideological motivation or rational argumentation of the human sciences, to bring about a new fundamental freedom in an institution based on the suppression of rights. In the meantime, the manifest achievements of UVF in terms of maintaining family ties and conjugal sexual relations remain a prerogative controlled and organized by the prison administration, which retains control over the occurrences and spatio-temporal conditions of the practices, while recognizing factually and limitatively the notion of respect for intimacy. In view of the conditions under which UVFs are granted, and the very small number of establishments equipped with this system, making sexuality possible remains an exceptional measure that constitutes both a release from frustrations and an intrusion by the institution into the management of intimacy. Undoubtedly, the recurrent intentions to normalize prison life, by analogy with life on the outside, obey severe and limited contingencies. The problem of monosexual confinement and control over the appropriateness of sexual relations will remain inherent to prison reality, which we know can never be organized on the basis of large-scale co-education, nor of respect for sexuality as a fundamental right.

---

310. The Regional Intervention and Security Teams (ERIS) were created in 2003. Their mission is "to ensure optimum security in prisons, by preventing escapes, mutinies, assaults on staff, suicides and prison violence". This new security unit is over-armed like a commando unit, and the violence of its "particularly muscular" interventions is of great concern to prisoners' associations.

EPILOGUE

Time to choose

The lack of sexual freedom hardly argues in favor of civic recognition of those whom the justice system of a democratic country has decided to exclude from society. This conception of confinement contributes to the stigmatization of individuals, which runs counter to the project of rehabilitation expressed in texts and speeches. Despite the limits of the system and the perversions that result from it, the advent of the Family Visiting Units is nonetheless a step in the direction of seeking coherence between a punitive system and the ambition for resocialization that underpins it. Either prison is a repressive penal tool, acting on the body, mind and legal attributes of individuals, in the total absence of any redemptive effect and in disregard of fundamental rights; the prohibition of sexuality is then self-evident, since the aim is to punish, or even avenge. Or democracy focuses on a more elaborate conception of prison, to ward off danger and reform people, in which case any denial of the most elementary rights, such as privacy, undermines a system that has already been defined as imperfect for centuries.

Prison doesn't invent new sexual situations. Detention simply reveals desires, practices and tastes, some of them repressed, whose disinhibition in prison is due to the contingency of confinement, gender uniqueness, discipline, and a general *lack of everything*. This is as true of homosexual practices as it is of the intense use of pornography or sexual accessories. Generally speaking, conditions of confinement exacerbate human temperaments, which find ways to survive the hostility of long sentences through adaptation mechanisms. Many sexual practices in prison are those of the *starving*, ready to break with a definition of personal dignity that no longer holds sway inside. The strength of the *ego* is measured by its ability to resist the pain of frustration, and the control of pleasure in general.

Imprisonment is fundamentally built on a principle of distancing people from each other. This suffering is inflicted without any real calculation, and while some of the inmates come out of it with serenity, often thanks to outside support that helps them to overcome their solitude, others dread being wounded for life. Through the regime it imposes, the prison organizes a distinction between those inmates who will resist as the years go by, and those who will regress, become corrupted, lose their self-esteem, and finally re-apprehend society on the outside with a hatred matched only by the self-loathing imprinted by imprisonment on their destiny. These are the "techniques of the self"[311], referred to by Michel Foucault, that are thwarted here, the consequences of which are to be considered in the light of the duration and respective capacities of each individual to bear the frustrations. Maintaining affective ties and communication with the outside world are fundamental to mitigating the rupture between inside and outside. The regime of constrained bodies and frustrated pleasures thus acts, on the basis of social and

---

311. "It is through the 'techniques of the self' that Foucault shows that the individual has recognized himself as the subject of a sexuality: these techniques constitute a certain relationship to oneself and to others, determine operations on oneself, on one's body, on one's soul, ways of behaving, being and transforming oneself in order to 'reach a certain state of happiness, purity, wisdom, perfection or immortality'." See FOUCAULT (Michel), DEFERT (Daniel) and EWALD (François), (eds.), "Les techniques de soi", in *Dits et écrits. 1980-1988*, Paris, Gallimard, 1994, p. 785.

psychological parameters, in a process of *natural selection* described here as *prison Darwinism.*

Considering that socialization is built and nurtured more than it is acquired, the prison institution and society must create the conditions to make living together a possibility, until it becomes self-evident in the majority of situations. This is the price of eradicating violence, fear, persistent divisions, injustice and all the circumstances that underlie and motivate crime and disorder. The danger of normalizing policies lies in the use of penalties as a substitute for the daily and eternal efforts that all of us, absolutely all of us, in an increasingly heterogeneous society, must make to build, conduct and maintain a social space in which everyone has their place.

The sexual experience of *long prison sentences is* akin to intense misery: the misery of pleasure, the misery of otherness, and the misery of subjects tortured by humiliation. Before being a deprivation of freedom, prison organizes a deprivation of otherness, understood as a fundamental constituent of life in society. In this emotional and sexual desert, survival is organized around marginal behaviors and perverse attitudes that would be frightening if indulgence and understanding of the specific contingencies of detention did not soften everyone's judgment. Confinement is destabilizing because of the loss of reference points. Unless the psyche is particularly well structured, it is illusory to expect prisoners to *redeem themselves* after years of detention.

Between the protection of society and the *punishment-amendment* process, the choice of penal policies is clear. The primary focus is on the outside world, which is victorious in terms of political concerns. Imprisonment remains an exception, mainly reserved for a category of individuals who, through their offence, underline a largely divided social allegiance, determined by common social, economic and cultural parameters. Faced with this reality, which is often ignored by the public and absent from political discourse, democracy must be vigilant. Initiatives to humanize prisons must not lead to the creation behind their walls of a veritable existence of relegation, through a long period of ostracism that will be alleviated thanks to the advent of new prerogatives such as UVF, or *improved* conditions of *comfort* in future detention centers. Whatever the new arrangements, the institution must never forget that reconstituting a portion of the outside world inside will never be the same as the gradual resocialization permitted by furloughs. The virtual is not and never will be the real. Penal policies aimed at mitigating the rupture between inside and outside, however essential they may be in the fight against recidivism and the reintegration of prisoners, cannot be understood without extreme vigilance with regard to the over-massive use of the principle of imprisonment, and with regard to the inevitable questioning of the progressive lengthening of sentences. Whatever its evolution, particularly in sexual matters, imprisonment remains an instrument of repression and domination. With a more humane prison, the temptation to lock people up *longer* and for longer is great. Thus, under the guise of *utilitarian generosity* towards a stigmatized penal population, the Republic would only become harsher, more oppressive and more unjust. But when it comes to prisons, it's undeniably and definitively a question of justice. It's worth remembering that, in line with European ambitions, prison is seen as a punitive solution of last resort. That's why reason dictates that it should be used sparingly. Unless politicians openly explain the half-spoken, half-spoken reality that even today, society legitimizes physical and psychological suffering as the ideal punishment, with arguments alternating between presumed effectiveness and regulated social vengeance.

Bibliography

AGRET (Roland), *L'Amour enchristé. Lettre ouverte à Élisabeth Guigou, garde des Sceaux et ministre de la Justice*, Paris, Blanche, 1998.

ALLEN (T.E.), "Psychiatric Observations on an Adolescent Inmate Social System and Culture", *Psychiatry*, vol. XXXII, no. 3, August 1969, pp. 292-302.

ALVAREZ (Josefina), "Chronique de l'exécution des peines", *Revue de sciences criminelles et de droit pénal comparé*, Paris, July-September 2006.

ARENDT (Hannah), *Condition of Modern Man*, Paris, Calmann-Lévy, 1983.

- *The Origins of Totalitarianism*, Paris, Le Seuil, 1998.

ARTIÈRES (Philippe) and LAÉ (Jean-François), *Lettres perdues, écriture, amour et solitude. XIXᵉ-XXᵉ siècles*, Paris, Hachette Littératures, 2003.

ASSEMBLÉE NATIONALE, MERMAZ (Louis), (chairman, FLOCH (Jacques), (rapporteur), Commission d'enquête sur la situation dans les prisons françaises, "La France face à ses prisons", rapport n° 2521, Paris, 2000, tome I (report, 328 pages) and tome II (hearings, 565 pages).

AUBERT (Nicole), ENRIQUEZ (Eugène), GAULEJAC (Vincent DE), *Le Sexe du pouvoir. Femmes, hommes et pouvoir dans les organisations*, Paris, Desclée de Brouwer, 1986.

AUZENET (Philippe), *Quand la justice nous casse*, Paris, Le Sarment/Fayard, 2001.

BAUMAN (Zygmunt), *L'Amour liquide. De la fragilité des liens entre les hommes*, Rodez, Le Rouergue/Chambon, 2004.

BENTHAM (Jeremy), *Panoptique*, Paris, Imprimerie nationale, 1791.

- *Traité de législation civile et pénale*, Paris, Rey et Gravier, 1830, tome II.

BETTELHEIM (Bruno), *The Conscious Heart. Comment garder son autonomie et parvenir à l'accomplissement de soi dans une civilisation de masse*, Paris, Robert Laffont, coll. "Réponses", 1972.

BORRILLO (Daniel), *L'Homophobie*, Paris, PUF, "Que sais-je?" collection, 2000.

- Liberté érotique et exception sexuelle", *in* BORRILLO (Daniel) and LOCHAK (Danièle), (eds.), *La Liberté sexuelle*, Paris, PUF, 2005.

BOUCARD (Robert), *Les Dessous des prisons de femmes*, Paris, Éditions de France, 1930.

BOUGEARD (Nathalie), *Lien social*, no 826, Paris, February 1st, 2007.

BOURDIEU (Pierre), *La Domination masculine*, Paris, Le Seuil, 1998.

BOZON (Michel), "Observer l'inobservable. La description et l'analyse de l'activité sexuelle", *in* BAJOS (Nathalie) *et al*, (sous la direction de), *Sexualité et sida*, Paris, Agence nationale de recherches sur le sida, December 1995.

BOZON (Michel), *Sociologie de la sexualité*, Paris, Armand Colin, 2005.

BUFFARD (Simone), *Le Froid pénitentiaire. L'impossible réforme des prisons*, Paris, Le Seuil, coll. "Esprit", 1973.

BURSTEIN (Jules Quentin), *Conjugal Visits in Prison*, Massachusetts/Toronto, Lexington books/D.C. Heath and Company Lexington, 1977.

BUTLER (Judith) and RUBIN (Gayle S.), *Marché au sexe*, Paris, Epel, 2001.

CARDON (Carole), "Relations conjugales en situation carcérale", *Ethnologie française*, "Intimités sous surveillance", vol. XXXII, no 1, Paris, PUF, January-March 2002.

CASTA-ROSAZ (Fabienne), *Histoire de la sexualité en Occident*, Paris, La Martinière, 2004.

CHANET (Laurence), "Prisons. Du droit à la sensualité et à la tendresse... à la mixité", *Actes*, nos. 45-46, Paris, June 1984.

CHARMES (Claude), *Le Maximum*, Paris, Stock, 1974.

CHAUVENET (Antoinette), ORLIC (Françoise), BENGUIGUI (Georges), *Le Monde des surveillants de prison*, Paris, PUF, coll. "Sociologies", 1994.

CHRISTIE (Nils), *L'Industrie de la punition. Prison and penal policy in the West*, Paris, Autrement, 2003. First edition, Crime Control as Industry. Towards Gulags, Oslo, Western Style, Universitetsforlaget, 1993.

COMBESSIE (Philippe), *Prisons des villes et des campagnes*, L'Atelier, coll. "Champs pénitentiaires", Paris, 1996.

- *Sociologie de la prison*, Paris, La Découverte, "Repères" series, 2001.

- "Surveillants de prison. Condamnés à l'obscurité?", *Informations sociales*, no 82, Paris, 2000.

European Committee for the Prevention of Torture and Inhuman or Degrading Treatment or Punishment (CPT), *Report to the Government of the French Republic by the CPT*, Brussels, January 19, 1993.

CORRAZE (Jacques), *L'Homosexualité*, Paris, PUF, "Que sais-je?" collection, 2000.

DANET (François) and FERRUCCI (Sophie), "Le projet de création d'"UVF' en prison verra-t-il le jour?", *Forensic*, nos. 7-8, Paris, September-December 2001.

DAOUST (Valérie), *De la sexualité en démocratie. L'individu libre et ses espaces identitaires*, Paris, PUF, 2005.

DESCARTES (René), *The Passions of the Soul*, Paris, Flammarion, 1996.

DESPREZ (Édouard), *De l'abolition de l'emprisonnement*, Paris, Dentu, 1868.

DILS (Patrick), *Je voulais juste rentrer chez moi... Un innocent 15 ans en prison*, Paris, Michel Lafon, 2002.

DOMENACH (Élise), "Quels sont nos droits et nos responsabilités face à l'expression pornographique?", *Cités*, no 15, Paris, PUF, 2003.

DORLÉANS (Annick), "Droit de la famille et détention", *Prison-justice*, no. 93, Paris, April 2001.

DUMONT (Étienne), *Théorie des peines et des récompenses*, Paris/London, Bossange et Masson, 1818, volumes I and II.

DÜNKEL (Frieder) and SNACKEN (Sonja), *Les Prisons en Europe*, Paris, L'Harmattan, coll. "La Justice au quotidien", 2005.

EIGENBERG (Helen M.), "Homosexuality in Male Prisons. Demonstrating the Need for a Social Constructionist Approach", *Criminal Justice Review*, February 17, 1992.

ELIAS (Norbert), *Engagement et distanciation*, Paris, Fayard, 1983.

ENRIQUEZ (Eugène) and HAROCHE (Claudine), *La Face obscure des démocraties modernes*, Ramonville Saint-Agne, Érès, coll. "Sociologie clinique", 2002.

ERIBON (Didier), "Ce que l'injure me dit. Quelques remarques sur le racisme et la discrimination", in *L'Homophobie. Comment la définir, comment la combattre*, Paris, Prochoix, 1999.

313

- *Réflexions sur la question gay*, Paris, Fayard, 1999.

FALCONNET (Georges) and LEFAUCHEUR (Nadine), *La Fabrication des mâles*, Paris, Le Seuil, 1975.

FAUGERON (Claude) and LE BOULAIRE (Jean-Michel), *Prisons and prison sentences*, Paris, CESDIP, 1991.

FLEURY (Élisabeth), *Le Parisien*, Paris, May 9, 2003.

FOUCAULT (Michel), *Dits et écrits. 1954-1988*, Paris, Gallimard, coll. "Quarto", 2001.

- *Histoire de la folie à l'âge classique*, Paris, Gallimard, 1961.

- *History of Sexuality I. La volonté de savoir*, Paris, Gallimard, 1976.

- *Histoire de la sexualité II. L'usage des plaisirs*, Paris, Gallimard, "Tel" series, 1984.

- *Histoire de la sexualité III. Le souci de soi*, Paris, Gallimard, 1984.

- *Les Mots et les Choses*, Paris, Gallimard, 1966.

- *Surveiller et Punir. Naissance de la prison*, Paris, Gallimard, 1975.

FRENCH (L.), "Prison Sexualization. Inmate Adaptation to 'Psycho-sexual Stress'", *Corrective and Social Psychiatry and Journal of Behaviour Technology, Methods and Theory*, vol. XXV, no. 2, 1979.

FREUD (Sigmund), *Abrégé de psychanalyse*, Paris, PUF, coll. "Bibliothèque de psychanalyse", 1975.

- "Des types libidinaux", in *Œuvres complètes*, Paris, PUF, 1995.

- *Inhibition, symptom and anguish*, Paris, PUF, 1993.

FROMM (Erich), *The Art of Loving*, Paris, Desclée de Brouwer, 1995.

GALOPIN (Arnould), *Les Enracinées*, Paris, Fayard, 1902.

GENET (Jean) and SARTRE (Jean-Paul), *Saint Genet. Comédien et martyr*, Paris, Gallimard, 1988.

GENET (Jean), "Miracle de la rose", in *Œuvres complètes*, Paris, Gallimard, 1972.

- *Journal du voleur*, Paris, Gallimard, 1949.

GODELIER (Maurice), "La sexualité est autre chose qu'elle-même", *Esprit*, Paris, March-April 2001.

- *L'Idéel et le Matériel. Pensée, économies, sociétés*, Paris, Fayard, 1984.

GOFFMAN (Erving), *Asiles. Études sur la condition sociale des malades mentaux*, Paris, Éditions de Minuit, 1968.

- *Stigmate. Les usages sociaux des handicaps*, Paris, Éditions de Minuit, coll. "Le Sens commun", 1975.

GONIN (Daniel), *La Santé incarcérée*, Paris, L'Archipel, 1991.

GRAVIER (Bruno) and LAMOTHE (Pierre), "La sexualité en prison: un comportement à risque?", paper presented at the 5th International AIDS Conference, Montreal, June 4-9, 1989.

HERZOG-EVANS (Martine), "Aspects juridiques de la sexualité des détenus en France", *Revue internationale de criminologie et de police technique et scientifique*, no 2, Geneva, April-June 2001.

- *La Gestion du comportement du détenu*, Paris, L'Harmattan, coll. "Logiques juridiques", 1998.

HOGGART (Richard), *The Culture of the Poor*, Paris, Éditions de Minuit, 1970.

ILLICH (Yvan), *La Convivialité*, Paris, Le Seuil, 1973.

INIZAN (Juliette), DEVEAUX (Solenne), VÊTU (Jean-Jacques), *Surveillantes en détention hommes*, Paris, Direction de l'administration pénitentiaire, T&D, 2002.

JACKSON (Bruce), *Their prisons. Autobiographies of American prisoners and ex-prisoners*, Paris, Plon, coll. "Terre humaine", 1975.

KANT (Emmanuel), *Anthropologie du point de vue pragmatique*, Paris, Flammarion, 1993, tome III.

LACAN (Jacques), *Travaux et interventions*, Alençon, AREP, 1977.

LAMBERT (Christophe), *Derrière les barreaux*, Paris, Michalon, 1999.

LAQUEUR (Thomas), *Le Sexe en solitaire*, translated from English by Pierre-Emmanuel Dauzat, Paris, Gallimard, 2005.

LE CAISNE (Léonore), *Prison. Une ethnologue en centrale*, Paris, Odile Jacob, 2000.

LEONARD (Jacques), "Les médecins des prisons", in PETIT (Jacques-Guy), (sous la direction de), *La Prison, le bagne et l'histoire*, Genève, Librairie des Méridiens, 1984.

LESAGE DE LA HAYE (Jacques), *La Guillotine du sexe. La vie affective et sexuelle des prisonniers*, Paris, L'Atelier/Éditions Ouvrières, 1998.

- *La Sortie de prison. Docker et psychologue*, Paris, Lesage de La Haye, 1981.

- *L'Homme de métal*, Paris, Existences, 1995.

LHUILIER (Dominique), RIDEL (Luc), SIMONPIETRI (Aldona), VEIL (Claude), *Identité professionnelle, identité de sexe et sida. Le cas des surveillants de prison*, Laboratoire de psychologie clinique, Université Paris VII, March 1998.

LHUILIER (Dominique) and AYMARD (Nadia), *L'Univers pénitentiaire. Du côté des surveillants de prison*, Paris, Desclée de Brouwer, coll. "Sociologie clinique", 1997.

LHUILIER (Dominique), "Intimité et sexualité des femmes incarcérées", in *La Lettre du Genepi*, Paris, Genepi, September-November 2003.

LINDNER (Robert M.), *Sex in Prison*, Fall, Complex, 1951.

LOCHAK (Danièle), "La liberté sexuelle, une liberté (pas) comme les autres?", *in* BORRILLO (Daniel) and LOCHAK (Danièle), (eds.), *La Liberté sexuelle*, Paris, PUF, 2005.

MANAUD-BENAZERAF (Sylvie), *Les Unités de visites familiales. Nouvelles pratiques, nouveaux liens*, Agen, Cirap, 2006.

MARCHETTI (Anne-Marie), *Perpétuités. Le Temps infini des longues peines*, Paris, Plon, coll. "Terre humaine", 2001.

MERMAZ (Louis) and FLOCH (Jacques), *La France face à ses prisons*, Paris, Assemblée nationale, coll. "Les Documents d'information de l'Assemblée nationale", 2000.

MINISTÈRE DE LA JUSTICE, *Rapport du groupe de travail sur la mise en œuvre des UVF*, Paris, June 1995.

MONNEREAU (Alain), *La Castration pénitentiaire. Droit à la sexualité pour les personnes incarcérées*, Paris, Lumière et justice, 1986.

MONTANDON (Cléopâtre) and CUETTAZ (Bernard), *Paroles de gardiens, paroles de détenus. Bruits et silences de l'enfermement*, Genève, Masson, coll. "Déviance et société", 1981.

MORRIS (Desmond), *De Naakte Aap*, Antwerp, Bruna en Zoon, 1968.

NIETZSCHE (Friedrich), *Beyond Good and Evil*, Paris, Aubier, 1978.

- *Œuvres philosophiques complètes*, texts and variants edited by G. Colli and M. Montinari, 14 volumes in 18 vols, Paris, Gallimard, 1967-1997.

O'BRIEN (Patricia), *Correction ou châtiment*, Paris, PUF, coll. "Les Chemins de l'histoire", 1988.

ONFRAY (Michel), *9 m²*, Paris, Le Cadratin/Actes Sud, 2006.

PETIT (Jacques-Guy), *Histoire des galères, bagnes et prisons*, Toulouse, Privat, 1991.

Pichot (Pierre) and Danjon (Suzanne), *Le Test de frustration de Rosenzweig*, Paris, Centre de psychologie appliquée, 1966.

Plato, *Le Banquet*, Paris, Flammarion, 1964.

Proust (Marcel), *Du côté de chez Swann*, Paris, Gallimard, "Folio" series, 1988.

Rabouin (David), *Le Désir*, Paris, Flammarion, "Corpus" series, 1997.

Rambourg (Cécile), *Les Unités de visites familiales. Nouvelles pratiques, nouveaux liens*, foreword by Sylvie Manaud-Benazeraf, Agen, Cirap, 2006.

Ricordeau (Gwénola), "Enquête sur l'homosexualité et les violences sexuelles en détention", *Déviance et société*, vol. XXVIII, no. 2, Geneva, June 2002.

- *La Solidarité familiale à l'épreuve de l'incarcération. Une analyse comparative*, Mission de recherche Droit et Justice, Paris, GIP, 2003.

Rostaing (Corinne), *La Relation carcérale. Identités et rapports sociaux dans les prisons de femmes*, PUF, coll. "Le Lien social", Paris, 1997.

Rousseau (Jean-Jacques), *Julie ou la Nouvelle Héloïse*, Paris, Flammarion, 1967.

- *Émile*, in *Œuvres complètes*, Paris, Gallimard, "Bibliothèque de la Pléiade" series, 1990.

Rubin (Gayle S.), *Penser le sexe. Pour une théorie radicale de la politique de la sexualité*, Paris, Epel, 2001.

Sabo (Don), Kupers (Terry A.), London (Willie), *Prison Masculinities*, Philadelphia, Temple University Press, 2001.

Schachtel (Martine), *Femmes en prison. Dans les coulisses de Fleury-Mérogis*, Paris, Albin Michel, 2000.

Schilder (Paul), *L'Image du corps*, Paris, Gallimard, 1968.

Seyler (Monique), *La Prison immobile*, Paris, Centre de recherches sociologiques sur le droit et les institutions pénales, 1990.

Spurk (Jan), *Quel avenir pour la sociologie*, Paris, PUF, 2006.

Stoller (Robert J.), *L'Excitation sexuelle. Dynamique de la vie érotique*, Paris, Payot, 1984.

- *L'Imagination érotique telle qu'on l'observe*, Paris, PUF, 1989.

Swinnen (E.), "La sexualité en prison, la visite conjugale et la prison mixte dans les pays américains", *Bulletin de l'administration pénitentiaire belge*, Belgium, January-February-March 1982.

- "La sexualité en prison, le régime de célibat en prison", *Bulletin de l'administration pénitentiaire belge*, Belgium, October-November-December 1981.

Sykes (Gresham M.), *The Society of Captives. A Study of a Maximum Security Prison*, Princeton (N.J.), Princeton University Press, 1958.

Tartakowsky (Pierre), *La Prison. Enquête sur l'administration pénitentiaire*, Paris, Payot/Rivages, "Documents Payot" series, 1995.

Théry (Irène), "La côte d'Adam. Retour sur le paradoxe démocratique", *Esprit*, no 273, Paris, March-April 2001.

Thomas Aquinas (Saint), *Summa Theologica*, Paris, Desclée et Cie, 1949.

Tocqueville (Alexis de), "Rapport à la Chambre des députés", *in* Beaumont (Gustave) and Tocqueville (Alexis de), *Le Système pénitentiaire aux États-Unis*, Paris, Gosselin, third edition, 1845.

Touraine (Alain), *Pourrons-nous vivre ensemble? Égaux et différents*, Paris, Fayard, 1998.

Veil (Claude) et Lhuilier (Dominique), (sous la direction de), *La Prison en changement*, Ramonville Saint-Agne, Érès, coll. "Trajet", 2000.

Wacquant (Loïc), "La prison est une institution hors la loi", *R de réel*, no 3, April 2000.

Wacquant (Loïc), *Les Prisons de la misère*, Paris, Raisons d'agir, 1999.

Welzer-Lang (Daniel), *Le Viol au masculin*, Paris, L'Harmattan, coll. "Logiques sociales", 1988.

Welzer-Lang (Daniel) and Mathieu (Lilian), "Des significations de la sexualité en milieu carcéral", *Les Cahiers de la sécurité intérieure*, "Prisons en société", no. 31, Paris, 1998.

- *Rapport de groupe de travail sur la mise en œuvre des UVF*, Paris, Ministère de la Justice, June 1995.

Welzer-Lang (Daniel), Faure (Mickaël), Mathieu (Lilian), *Sexualités et violences en prison*, Lyon, OIP/Aléas, 1996.

Table of contents

SECOND PART
LIVING YOUR SEXUALITY IN PRISON - *The missing otherness -*

THIRD PART
TENTATIONS AND DANGERS OF CARCERAL HOMOSEXUALITY
- Otherness forbidden -

Table of contents

PART FIVE
THE THWARTED AMBITIONS OF REINTEGRATION

EPILOGUE
Time to choose

Best sellers Max Milo Editions

Hitler's banker, Jean-François Bouchard

Confessions of a forger, Éric Piedoie Le Tiec

The Koran and the flesh, Ludovic-Mohamed Zahed

Governing by fake news, Jacques Baud

Governing by chaos, Collectif

A political history of food, Paul Ariès

Mad in U.S.A.: The ravages of the "American model",
Michel Desmurget

Mondial soccer club geopolitics, Kévin Veyssière

Putin: Game master?, Jacques Braud

Treatise on the three impostors: Moses, Jesus, Muhammad,
The Spirit of Spinoza

TV Lobotomy, Michel Desmurget